The Technique Of Rest

Anna Callender Brackett

THE TECHNIQUE
OF REST

BY

ANNA C. BRACKETT

As for Leisure
" The fashion of it men forgot
About the age of chivalry"

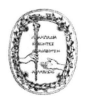

NEW YORK

HARPER AND BROTHERS

MDCCCXCIII

Copyright, 1892, by HARPER & BROTHERS.

"My roof is hardly picturesque—
It lacks the pleasant reddish brown
Of the tiled house-tops out of town,
And cannot even hope to match
The modest beauty of the thatch;
Nor is it Gothic or grotesque—
No gable breaks, with quaint design,
Its hard monotony of line,
And not a gargoyle on the spout
Brings any latent beauty out;
Its only charm—I hold it high—
Is just its nearness to the sky."

CONTENTS.

THE

TECHNIQUE OF REST

I

REST

THE occasion of this book is an article of mine in HARPER'S NEW MONTHLY MAGAZINE for June, 1891, called "The Technique of Rest," which was an attempt to help, out of my own rather wide experience, some of the women who were tired. From different parts of the country, and from women whom I had never heard of, came letters of thanks for the help given to

1

them—letters written evidently out of very full and very weary lives. Then it was suggested to me that more might be said on the same subject, for which there seemed to be a decided demand. Thanks and appreciation were universal from the women who spoke of the article ; it seemed to have touched the right chord, and for that I was very thankful, since the world of women is not destitute of effort, nor is its effort purposeless, but the purpose is too often methodless, and so, much brave effort is worse than wasted. This is particularly the case in home life, the demands of which must of necessity be multifarious and never-ending. Where woman has taken her place in business she has found her method ready-shaped for her, and following that, she does her work, if with a certain amount of monotony, yet without undue fatigue. Her hours are fixed, and as a rule she

gets needful change of scene as she
goes to her business and returns to her
home or the place where she lives.
But the "home-maker" has not, nor
can she have, any such change, and
her hours are always from the rising of
the sun beyond the going down of the
same. She cannot get away from the
demands made upon her, and as the
years go on, these tighten more and
more. She may try to escape them,
but they are more in number than the
sands of the sea, and disappear for a
moment only to return in other and
more complicated forms. The more
humble and the more in earnest she
grows, the more weary she gets, till she
lives in a perpetual sense of not being
able to draw one full breath. Many a
woman will recognize the truth of these
words, though it will seem to most men
that they are exaggerated. I said above
that from women I had received only

warm thanks and appreciation for my
words in the " Technique of Rest."   I
should add that I sent it to a man—a
psychologist—who said in return: " I
have read your article; it is good, but
too grim." That was not what the
women thought; they knew it was not
too grim for the truth.

It is sometimes asked why things in
the home cannot be regulated in the
same way as they are in business.   It
can be done to a certain but very limited extent, for to do more would destroy the very idea of a home.   Times
for meals can be maintained if the man
of the family does not make that impossible.   Beyond this regularity there
must be a large degree of flexibility
Peace and rest are the characteristics
of the home.   But it should not be a
peace which is only a stifled war, and
the Rest must come from the constant
balance of the complicated conditions,

yielding at every side with a certain
compensating movement, so that it
shall yet be firm and supporting. That
this is impossible is no reason why it
should not be accomplished. One is
reminded of Montaigne's saying that
only when a thing becomes incredible
is there any room for faith. A woman
has power to accomplish the impossible, and she should never fear to un-
dertake it. Just that she may do this
is she made so quick and so facile, so
able to turn from one thing to another,
and so sensitive to outside impressions.
Give her the width of information which
she lacks because of the narrowness of
her education, and she will free herself
from the coils which render her breath-
ing difficult, and find herself able to
create a home without, in doing it,
sacrificing herself. But in order to
do this, she must work from within,
outward; she must create within her-

self the strength which shall be equal
to that pressing upon her from without.
For it is only in a balance of forces
that Rest consists. It is not anything
in and for itself; it is only the harmony
of demand and supply, the supply varying as the demand varies, no matter
how often or how greatly, with the
beautiful sureness of some of the sewing machines.

What we want is an automatic tension attachment to every woman. Then
the work will run easily, and the stitches
will be of even length, even though the
pull be now strong and now weak. Rest
is not rust. It may at some times mean
the absolute do-nothingness longed for
by the old woman whose pathetic last
words I have never been able to divest,
my memory of since I first read them,
centuries ago. I am quite sure these
lines must have been written by a woman, though their authorship has never

yet been claimed to my knowledge.
What makes them pathetic is their unmistakable truth.   I give the epitaph :

" Here lies a poor woman who always was tired,
   For she lived in a house where help was not hired,
   Her very last words were, ' My friends, I am going
   To a place where there's nothing of washing or sewing !
   Oh, everything there will be just to my wishes,
   For where they don't eat, there's no washing of dishes.
   The courts with sweet anthems are constantly ringing,
   But having no voice, I shall get clear of singing !"
   She folded her hands with her latest endeavor,
   And whispered,' Oh, nothing, sweet nothing forever !' "

In the whole range of literature, I do
not think there is anything which can
match the eighth line for completeness
and finish of thought.   It is evident
that the question of the music had for
a time troubled her, but that the moment had come in which that anxiety
also had been dispelled, and she was
ready to fold her hands—another stroke
of genius — in perfect confidence that
at last there was no more doubt as to
the complete rest awaiting her.   It is

doubtless true that Nirvana offers great
attractions to many women, and that
the preacher who would strive to lead
them by picturing heaven as a place of
continual activity is misdirecting his
efforts.

In the same strain was the recent account of the suicide of a woman found
dead at eighty years old, in the house
of her grandson, where she was living.
Under her pillow there was a half-emp-
tied bottle of laudanum and a piece of
paper on which she had written, "This
will be the last time of my going to
bed." One can easily imagine the feeling of rest at last with which the poor
old woman wrote these words—a pro-
test against the deadly monotony of
daily existence, against the continual
drudgery of dressing and undressing,
which necessarily forms so large a part
of the duties of every day, and which,
whenever we become conscious of it, is

so wearily tiresome. Sometimes there is no other rest but absolute do-nothing, and therefore has a pitiful God made death a component part of every life, a something without which life would be incomplete. But this does not invalidate the statement made above, that Rest is in any case only harmony between the inside and the outside conditions of life. If these conditions be not harmonious, then one of them must be tuned up or down to the other. And this tuning cannot be done once for all, but must be a continual care. Every day brings its own conditions and new complications. The orchestra· cannot tune its instruments to last through even one concert. Always there must be new adjustments after every piece of music, and so it is with human life. That human nature is always wanting to embody its experience, whether religious or political, in

creeds and in laws is only a proof of
how it longs for rest; and the fact of
revision of creeds and laws shows also
that this effort is of no use except as
leading to a new activity. As Professor
James has so well said, the mere nam-
ing of anything gives us a certain sense
of rest and repose. It is as if we fastened the new idea with a label, and
now might reasonably hope that it
would cease tormenting us with its per-
sistent presence, and leave us free to
attend to other things. When Adam
had named all the animals, he must
have gone to sleep for the first time
with a quiet hope of undisturbed repose. It is very simple to name a
thing. To formulate a creed—that is,
to name a conviction on the profound-
est subject of thought—is a more difficult task, but really in the very same
line. To the questions which have
concerned us, we give a formal answer:

We say, "I am tired of being continually haunted by you. I believe exactly so and so and once for all. Now let me rest." And the Church does rest, but only for a while. Or the State says, "Let us decide forever, and in a way that no one can misunderstand, the question of what shall be considered crimes, and what punishments shall be allotted to the doers of these offences. We will settle all the problems of property so that any questions which can possibly arise shall be easily adjusted." And so it does, or tries to do. But a live world, whether of thought or of action, cannot be kept in such swaddling-clothes, so that the history of the world is only a story of perpetual revision in one region or another. When nations have fought till they are tired, they call for rest in the form of a treaty, and they hope that now, at last, there will be a final settlement of the

vexed questions. We are always hear-
ing about " final settlements," and it
takes us a considerable part of our lives
to comprehend that there is no such
thing as a final settlement of anything,
and that we need not look for it. Whether in large or in small affairs, there
must be perpetual readjustment. All
the monotony there really is, is a monotony of change, and this is no more
so in household affairs than in all others. Therefore, women ought not to
complain of monotony in their lives, as
if it were something especially belonging to them. It is the law of any live
universe. Neither ought they to expect that they can escape the need of
constant tuning.

Where the harmony between the inner desire and the outside circumstances
does not exist—in other words, where
there is no rest—the question to be settled is, first of all, which of the two is to

be changed. Five from ten does not leave eight, but we can get eight by changing five to two just as easily as by substituting thirteen for ten. There are always at least two ways of doing a thing, and there are generally more than two. The thoughtless person goes blindly to work, changing the first condition that presents itself to his view, though the fact that it does so present itself. may be a mere accident. But what we need is the breadth of mind which brings all the conditions before it, the clearness of sight which discriminates, weighs, and measures, and this with always present thought of the end to be attained or to be approached; and last, but not least, the cool self-control which poises untroubled with balanced wing over all the conditions, suspending action till a rational decision has been reached. Even the hawk does not descend over the lake where the ducks are swimming without doing all these things. To those who see what they imply, it will be clear why the *manner* of the education of the little girl who is to be confronted by all the complicated and ever-changing problems of home-creation is of far more consequence than *what* she is learning.

Rest you cannot compass till you have secured harmony of the internal and external conditions of your own life, whatever that life may be. The question is always which of these conditions you can change. It may be possible, of course, that both are capable of modification. If so, the problem becomes more complicated. If, however, you decide, after a careful review of all the outside circumstances, that they cannot be altered, then your task is to mould your own mind into harmony with those conditions. Every effort to do this will be an approximation towards Rest. But bear always in mind that this must be a perpetually active process, and keep your mind ever open to the appreciation of the changes of the outward world. Harmony is not a simple thing. If the bass changes, perhaps the soprano must also change, and perhaps, also, the contralto and the tenor. You are not dealing with dead matter, if there be indeed any such thing as dead matter in the universe of God. You are dealing with His live world on the one hand, and on the other with your own live soul, and the possibilities of combination are practically infinite. Therein lies the interest of the problem. And if you can bring yourself to look at it as a problem, a game which you have to play out and to be triumphant in, so much the better. There will then enter into it a certain keen intellectual zest which will be of great service. The less personal feeling and the more cool intellect you can throw into the game the better. If you could stand far enough off from the question which you have to solve, it would all become perfectly clear to you. If you could stand far enough off either in space or in time, it would be comparatively easy. You do not suppose that God has any difficulty in seeing clear through all the problems of His Providence, or that to Him any one event, no matter how small and insignificant in your eyes, can be troubled or interfered with by any other, no matter how great. It is true you have not His infinite sight, but you can get farther away than you are from the pressing problems of to-day and here, if you will make a determined effort. And the farther away you can get, the more they will fall into harmony. It is because the conditions lie so close before your eyes that you cannot see to disentangle them. Try in the freedom of your mind to withdraw from them by never so little a space, and the crossing and tangled lines will begin to weave into some kind of order. Necessity—that is, God and His world, the whole of it—stands outside of you. Within you, you have the freedom which God has given. It is your business to reconcile that necessity and that freedom, since it is only in such reconciliation that Rest can be found. Find it! It can be found thus, no matter how seemingly mean or how so-called monotonous is the round of your daily life. It is for every woman in her own life to lay out her own course to the desired haven, and, as a rule, she will find it easier to steer her own ship than to try to steer the heavenly bodies or change the currents of the ocean.

If your weariness is simply bodily exhaustion, then you need, for restoration, only bodily repose. But this is almost never the case with a grown-up wom-

2

an. Generally with her, the exhaustion comes from the mind. With children it is different. A child who is properly looked after, goes to sleep when it is tired, and wakes up refreshed and as good as new, for sleep is an unfailing restorative for mere bodily weariness, and in that case is sure to come to the rescue. Indeed, so long as you sleep well and eat well, you have no great reason to complain; but in the weariness arising from the mind, sleep is not so ready to come. The child may reach this trouble in the same way. The sensitive, conscientious child may be driven to it by being forced into introspection — a state which is not natural to the immature mind—or it may come to the child intellectually through bad teaching in school. Anything which produces want of harmony in the mind will bring nervous exhaustion in a greater or a less degree. When the conscience has been

freed, or when the difficulty has been
solved, the face will brighten and the
look of care disappear.

Over and over again, Rest consists
simply in producing harmony between
the individual and her surroundings or
the conditions under which she has to
live. This harmony must be created by
herself, for when God created us in His
own image He could not do otherwise
than to make us active agents, and to or-
dain that if we wanted anything, we must
get it for ourselves. You cannot teach
the child by forcing facts upon him; so
long as you do this, they remain foreign
to him. It is only the knowledge that
he himself actively takes in and assim-
ilates till it becomes a part of his being
that goes towards his education. He
himself must reach out actively for it
or it can never become his. It is so
with Rest. It cannot be pasted on to
us nor forced down into our minds or

hearts. We must reach out and take it. In the case of affliction or trouble, where rest will not come till real resignation comes, we might at first think that it could be passively obtained, but this is so far from being the case that no greater effort could be required of us than to put our minds into the passive state requisite for being worked upon. Did you ever try to hear the sound of the crickets in the summer twilight and find yourself unable to do so, simply because your ear was tuned to the rustle of the poplar leaves or to the twitter of the birds? In such case a strong and vigorous effort is required to tune down the ear to the chirping, and only then is it borne in upon you, though you were surrounded by it all the time. Just so there is always plenty of Rest lying all round you, eager to press in and take possession of you, but you must take and control the other things with a

steady· and sometimes with a forceful
hand before it can reach you. This is
true. Believe it, if you do not know it,
for the belief that it is so will be one
great step towards the knowledge of it.

" ' Oh, where is the sea ?' the fishes cried,
　　As they swam the crystal clearness through ;
　' We've heard from of old of the ocean's tide,
　　And we long to look at the waters blue.
　The wise ones speak of the infinite sea ;
　Oh, who can tell us if such there be ?'

　The lark flew up in the morning bright,
　　And sung and balanced on sunny wings ;
　And this was its song : ' I see the light,
　　I look o'er a world of beautiful things ;
　But flying and singing everywhere,
　In vain I have searched to find the air.' "

This is too often the case. Before
" Thy will be done," came the sorrow
and the heaviness, and so they come
still in America as well as in Palestine.
Resignation is not merely a passive
state. It is an intensely active one in

which the soul is standing on tiptoe
"with arms out-stretched and eager
face ablaze." If conditions cannot be
changed, then they must be submitted
to, but not after the manner of the Ma-
hometan sailor who drops upon the
deck when the wind rises, refusing to
try to handle the ship because Allah
will save him in any case if it be His
will, and he will be destroyed in spite of
all his efforts if Allah has so ordained
it. We are not Orientals, and Allah is
not the name of our God. The freedom
the Orient has never known and can
never know is ours, but only for a great
price, and that price, our own effort.
Our place is not with the sailors who,
when the ship took fire, "leaped and
left her," but with those who "stood by
her, firing steady," as Helen Gray Cone
says, and it was only for them that the
old sailor in the tale invoked rest. You
must have trust in Someone else than

yourself, and in a wiser Sight than your
own. If you have not this trust, you
must fight for it till you win it. Sometimes the people who claim to love God
most, trust Him least. They seem unwilling to leave anything to Him, as if
He were incompetent. They insist upon
trying to do the work of His world-
currents as if these were of no avail,
and when great events happen they as-
sume to stand as His interpreters, or
they talk of " mysteries " as if they expected to fathom His counsels! They
make the mistake of trying to comprehend the Infinite. Although presumably
they have read the book of Job, they
talk as if in the kingdom of God we
were in a market-place, where articles
were laid out openly for sale, and where
we could buy anything, if only we were
willing to pay what we consider its fair
price in any coin which might happen
to be most convenient for us, unmind-

ful of the coinage of the kingdom. We must not expect to buy with Cæsar's coins any other than the goods of Cæsar. In the first place, we must hold to Montaigne's teaching—that it is only when we meet an incredible thing that there is any occasion at all for faith. In the second place, we must know that it is with the heart and never with the intellect "that man believeth unto righteousness," and that it is the pure in heart, and not the keen in intellect, who shall see God. "Mere intellectual reasoning will never lead to the knowledge of divine things;" and we must try to see that "demonstrative evidence which left no room for doubt would be absolutely fatal to any morality, because it would leave no place for faith or deliberate choice." It is from a critique in the London *Spectator* on the poems of Robert Browning that I am quoting, where the writer says that Browning

knew, and insisted upon it, that "purity
of heart and loyal love were the only
sure avenues to the knowledge of God
and His ways." "Eternal failure is the
only condition of spiritual progress."
We must, first of all, understand the
principle of the spiritual harvest, and
cease to expect to reap money or fine
clothes from good deeds. This, to begin with, will free us from much unrest.

Those who by daily living have in
some degree attained this insight have
no reason to be troubled over any failure
in memory which advancing age may
bring. Emily Dickinson wisely asks,
"Is it oblivion *or absorption* when things
pass from our minds?" We take out
our watch to look at the time in order
to decide whether we will follow some
course of action. We decide, and put
the watch back again, and are perhaps
troubled afterwards to find that we cannot remember what the time was. But

that was not what we wanted to know;
what we did want to know was whether
we should or should not do a certain
thing.   The knowledge of the exact
hour was only a means to an end; we
ought to be glad that we do not remember it.   Of what avail would it be to be
able to recite, never so perfectly, the
bills of fare of the meals which have
nourished us?   We don't want to remember such things; we want to have
forgotten them.   This is the case with
much of our knowledge also; we do
not want to hold it in our minds.   We
want to have read a certain book, but
we do not need to remember the con-
tents of the book.   It is the results
which we have garnered that are of
consequence to us, not the steps by
which we attained them.   It is what
we *are*, not what we have done, or what
any one else has done, that concerns us.
If our lives have been worth anything,

they have given us some degree of insight, which is only a sort of mental instinct telling us at once what to do
under certain conditions, just as we in-
voluntarily close our eyes if a blow be
aimed at our faces, or throw out our
arms if we slip on the ice.   There is a
theory, not at all improbable, that what
is known as instinct in the race is only
the gathered and assimilated wisdom
of all our ancestors.   In the same way,
the insight which comes with advancing age, and which makes the advice of
its possessors valuable, is only the gradually assimilated wisdom gained from
long years in which we have been forced
to reason out many problems, and to
contemplate with more or less satisfac-
tion the results of innumerable deeds,
whether our own or those of others.
The remembrance of those deeds, these
courses of action and their results, have
been generalized in the mind, till now,

when we are asked a question on any
subject with which we are familiar,
we see at once without conscious reasoning the way of action which it would
be probably best to adopt.   People say
sometimes after asking for advice, "But
you do not think about the thing at all!
I wanted to talk it over with you," not
realizing that we have been doing nothing else but thinking about that very
thing and a host of others of the same
nature all our lives, till we have only to
propose the question to the mind thus
trained, and the answer starts out like
the answer to a puzzle, or the result of
an arithmetical example in a calculating
machine.   It seems possible that the
gathered and assorted experiences of our
lives here are to become the instincts
of our life hereafter—the instincts with
which we shall start on that new life.
It may well be that we shall no longer remember any of the events or re-

flections which led to the formation
of those instincts, or shall only at times
dimly recall them as half-remembered
visions of some uncertain life beyond
our ken, retaining as material for our
new experiences only their results in
consciousness. Towards such a purpose the weakening, as it is called,
of mere memory as years go on seems
to point or dimly to hint. It certainly
is a method of action not inconsistent
with what we see and know of that God
before whom not one sparrow falls to
the ground unnoticed, and who in Nature is always teaching us the lesson of
how material worn out in one sort of
service is the fittest to employ in carrying out a different and a higher purpose. If there be one lesson more than
another taught by all study of natural
phenomena, it is that of this sort of
economy. There is no niggardliness
in the means employed to gain a cer-

tain end, or to carry out a previously
determined plan ; but after that plan
has been carried out, there is never any
waste of the smallest bit of material.
Always every fragment is taken up and
put to some new use "that nothing be
lost;" there was no more characteris-
tically divine saying than the direction
given by Christ after the miracle of the
loaves and fishes.

Let your memory transmute itself
into insight, passing into a higher and a
better thing. Waste no vain regrets over
it, and as to the flight of time, the hurry
and bustle of the swiftly recurring, the
swiftly vanishing days in which you
would do so much, and in which, it
seems to you, you can do so little, remember

" Yesterday, to-day, to-morrow come ;
    They hustle one another and they pass ;
  But all our hustling morrows only make
    One smooth to-day of God."

After all, every day which seems so
long and so hard to us is only a part
of the whole, and not a whole in itself;
and many a trouble and vexation, many
a thing hard to bear and difficult to
manage, will lose much of its importance in our eyes if we can stop to remember that it is only a part of a whole
which we cannot see, and a component
part of a smaller whole—the life given
to us. If we say, " It is only a part "
when it comes, and try to manage it as
such, we shall find that it is not totally
discouraging, and so can take hold of
it with more confidence and trust. We
are living not in a finished abode where
we might have reason to expect regularity and completeness, nay, not even
in a half-finished house, but really only

IN THE QUARRY.

Impatient, stung with 'pain and long delay,
I chid the roughhewn stone that round me lay;
I said—" What shelter art thou from the heat?
What rest art thou for tired and wayworn feet?

What beauty hast thou for the longing eye ?
Thou nothing hast my need to satisfy !"
And then the patient stone fit answer made—
" Most true, I am no roof with welcome shade;
I am no house for rest, or full delight
Of sculptured beauty for the weary sight ;
Yet am I still material for all ;
Use me as such—I answer to thy call ;
Nay, tread me only under climbing feet,
So serve I thee, my destiny complete ;
Mount by me into freer, purer air,
And find the roof that archeth everywhere ;
So what but failure seems, shall build success,
For all, as possible, thou dost possess."

Who by the Universal squares his life,
Sees but success in all its finite strife.
In all that is, his truth-enlightened eyes
Detect the May-be through its thin disguise ;
And in the Absolute's unclouded sun,
To him the two already are the one.

We are too apt to forget that all we
have now is only material.

Of one thing we may be sure : away
from rest, if that is what we are seek-
ing, or after which we are longing, lead
all small and petty thoughts, all mean-

ness and all narrow things, "pride,
vainglory and hypocrisy, envy, hatred,
and malice, and all uncharitableness."
The roads to it are by all great and
everlasting things, by humility, sinceri-
ty, truth, magnanimity, forgiveness, and
—in the noble and characteristic words
of ex-Senator Edmunds—that "inex-
tinguishable joy which comes from having been faithful to truth and self-re-
spect." When we have once found out
that

' 'Tis not the grapes of Canaan that repay,
  But the high faith that failed not by the
      way,"

we shall have found the place where
Rest dwells

3

II

NECESSITY

OME of us at least can remember the house-keeping
in old days, the extremest
demands of which, in spite
of the lapse of time, are still
to be found in our New England towns.
If we look at the work expected as a matter of course from many a farmer's wife
of to-day, we can only exclaim, "Who is
sufficient for these things?"   She is up
at four or five, and, finding perhaps her
fire made for her, prepares the breakfast, washes and dresses the children,
clears away the dishes, washes clothes,
puts the house to rights, takes care of
the milk, often of twenty cows, cleans
and dries the pans and makes the but-

ter. Meanwhile she is cooking the din-
ner for three or four hungry men and
serving it. Afterwards the dishes and
what a little friend of mine used to call
the "pot-pans" are to be washed and
cleared off, though she has learned to
put away nothing which is to be used
for the next meal, but to lay those dishes
and plates back on the table in preparation for supper when the "men-folks"
will be in from field work. The children are mostly taking care of themselves in some of the many places so
dear to the childish heart which a barn
and all sorts of sheds offer, though they
need intermittent attention and an ever-
watchful ear; then she mixes and bakes
hot biscuit for tea, and has everything
ready when the men-folks come, for
often they can't afford to waste a minute, having to return to the fields.
Then more dishes are to be washed
and the table must be set in readiness

for breakfast, the room cleaned, the
lamp lighted, the children put to bed
and the mending done, and so to sleep,
provided a summons do not come from
a neighboring farm-house that "My
woman is too sick to be left alone, and
I thought mebbe you would come in
and help us for to-night." And so it
goes on day after day in which all the
water that is used must be drawn, or at
the best, pumped outside the house,
brought into the kitchen, carried wherever it is needed, and then when used,
fetched out again, for in many a New
England house to-day the luxury of a
sink into which water can be poured is
unknown. It should not be forgotten,
either, that all this must be done without any helping hand. There is no
servant to take up the ends of the
work, such as to mop the floor after the
main work is done, or to blacken the
stove and "tidy up." No loose ends

can be left, for they would only make
more work for the next day, and that is
not to be thought of. It is no wonder
that the woman often looks forward
with a real sense of rest to the very
first weeks of the life of a new baby,
because she knows that for that time
at least, she can lie still and have some-
body else do the manual labor, if not
the thinking.

I do not mean that the husband has
been idle or neglectful. He, too, is
busy; but it is nevertheless true that
if there be an errand which necessitates
a " hitching up " of the horse and a
drive to the village, he is generally the
one to go, and thus at least he gets a
little change, and the sight of other people with different interests from those
on his own farm, while to the woman
there is no such respite except once in
a while the sewing-circle, which brings
with it more dishes to wash and more

cooking to do. Or if she takes the eggs—which in New England generally are, by an old traditional law, her perquisite—to the village to sell, or rather to barter, she often finds herself confronted with the hard problem of painfully trying to contrive how she can manage to make a dress out of a very small pattern of calico—all that she can get in exchange, after spending the necessary amount for her husband's tobacco. This is no exaggerated picture, as whoever will spend a summer in one of the back towns will learn, if he will take pains to become acquainted with the facts.

This story may sound strange and far away; but even in our cities fifty years ago, and with well-to-do families, all the water used had to be carried over the house; for the running water, even where it was found, would not run above the first floor, and scarcely there

on washing-days. All the dishes used
at meals had to be brought to the din-
ing-room from the kitchen on trays,
generally up a flight of stairs, and taken
back again in the same way afterwards.
Any woman who has done this work or
has seen it done, knows what an amount
of labor it involves, if not to the house-
keeper, then to the servants. Now we
have running water and waste-pipes all
over our houses; dumb-waiters for all
sorts of purposes, and more servants
than in those old days, and yet the
work of the house is never done, and
everybody is complaining of being tired.
The ways of living have been rendered
vastly easier by a multitude of inventions, by the increasing wealth of the
country, by better and more intelligent
service; and yet life is by no means
easier, but indeed harder. The demands on time, whether real or imag-
ined, have increased in a greater ratio

than the supply of facilities for answering them, and as the earth provokingly continues to revolve on its axis just as rapidly as of old, the days are never long enough for all the duties which they bring. It is as if everybody had had dealings with Andersen's Moor Woman, " a venomous old creature and never idle," who, among other industries, " sewed running leather to put into the shoes of human beings, so that they should never be at rest." The very existence of the conveniences increases the number of possible accidents, and of calls on our attention. The more complicated the structure of an animal, the more in number are the possible derangements of the parts of that structure — the more diseases it is liable to, and the more care must be spent to preserve health, or the more trained skill to restore it, if lost. Physicians multiply, and in the household the plumber's

bill may become one of the regular ex-
penses, as much as those of the grocer
and the butcher. The woman who has
seen water pouring out of her kitchen
range because the "water-back" has
burst during the night, and has considered the resemblance in complication of
the modern house to the human body,
has ceased to wonder at the curious
and almost incredible diseases which
may befall either. If she be not too
tired, she will look on, after that experience, with a sort of amused wonder
at what will happen next in a world
where all things seem possible, and
most of them probable. The care necessary in a modern house always re-
minds one of the poor man who could
never be perfectly dressed, because as
soon as he got a new hat his shoes began to wear out, and he hastily provided
himself with new shoes only to find
that his necktie was fraying, and so on

forever. If there be not something the matter with the roof, you may be sure that there is with the cellar, and if the warm-water faucet in the kitchen does not drip, the gas-burners need attention.

When we were little girls we could never succeed in "playing paper dolls." We were always cutting new dresses or hats for them in anticipation of entertainments which had no time to come off, because when they were all ready or almost ready for these great events, it grew dark, and it was time to put away our playthings and get ready for supper. It is very much the same with us now that we are only older children. We are always getting ready to live, and never having time enough to live. And by-and-by it begins to grow dark, and we must put up our playthings and go to bed. It is a pity, and there must be some way out of the mistake. Perhaps if we had not been so anxious to have

our dolls so variously arrayed, they
might have gone to more.parties, and
been happier dolls. But it is now too
late to restore to them anything of the
life which they lost, for they and their
dresses and hats have long ago van-
ished with the rest of our childish
treasures. What we might have done
for them and did not do, however, perhaps their memory may do for us, and
then their paper lives will not have
been in vain.

We go on multiplying our conveniences only to multiply our cares. We
increase our possessions only to the enlargement of our anxieties. There is, I
presume, no careful house-keeper who
has not, in some desperate moment of
going to the country or of returning
therefrom, wished that civilization had
never existed, and envied the freedom
of the Indian woman who could peace-
fully leave her wigwam to the prairie-

dogs and carry her wardrobe on her
back. But such wishes as these are
unavailing; we are living in modern
cities, and we must find some way out
of our own problems, not falling into
"blue-rose melancholy," which is of all
things the narrowest and the most hopeless. We are not alone in the trouble
forced upon us by the innumerable inventions, products of the intense mental activity of the time into which we
were born. All the comfort to be derived from the knowledge that we are
only a part of a large company, we
have. The old farmer, ruefully con-
templating his potato patch, says, "It
does somehow seem as if every time a
man invented a new machine to save
us work, the Lord invented a new bug!"
But as we can fight fire most successfully with fire, so we must fight the
army of inventions with our own. Build-
ings are not fire-proof unless they are

built of material that has had the fire
itself for godmother. To our own power of invention, therefore, we must turn
if we would not be overcome. The
spirit of the age, which has stimulated
the mental activity of other people, has
not left us untouched; and though it
seems sometimes as if it were an un-
equal fight with the whole world against
one woman, we may avail ourselves of
our quickened power of thinking to
create and utilize many little devices
which, though small in themselves, will
help not a little to smooth our way.

First among these may, perhaps, be
counted, increasing the elasticity of our
income. In our day, needs and desires
grow faster than the bank account. But
what we have is, after all, only the ratio
between the two, and not either by itself. If we can't increase the latter,
we have the ability to lessen the former,
and the result in peace of mind, and

consequently in power to battle cool-
ly and successfully with what we have
to do, will be just so much increased.
The suggesting of this might belong
as properly to the chapter on Freedom.
As an English writer says, "The great
thing in these circumstances is to avoid,
as much as possible, breaking into the
precious coins, and testing the resources
of what that clever woman, Ann Taylor
(Mrs. Gilbert), called the eminent firm,
Messrs. Hook, Crook & Co.   There
was once an upper servant, valuable in
many ways, who, when her new mis-
tress gave her an undergarment to patch
and the wherewithal to accomplish it,
observed, 'I will do my best, madam,
but I have never worn anything patched
myself.'   That young person never
found her income elastic, though she
lived to desire that it had been so, but
she did not go the right way to work.
It is mainly by judicious patching, mend-

ing, turning about, and the preserva-
tion of unconsidered trifles, that middle-
class incomes can be made elastic, and
the kind of life that consists of an end-
less succession of calls, afternoon teas,
and tennis tournaments does not con-
duce to it at all. The possessors of
narrow incomes should purchase wisely
and at fixed times, if they mean to make
the best of everything ; and if only they
have a little stock of ready cash to
start with, they can buy when and where
they see what suits them. By fixed times
we mean at the after - season summer
and winter sales, instead of starting out
to buy summer frocks in May and winter ones in October, when thin or thick
materials, as the case may be, are in
season. It is really very difficult to increase the purchasing power of money,
but time is money in the one sense that
time may be made to serve instead of
money ; and there are thousands of

families where breakfast is early, in order that the masculine portion may go to business, and the women have long, clear days before them in which to make the best of things, and yet can have the hour's reading or rest, or the occasional outing that redeems life from dulness, while the pleasure of proving that a given income can be made elastic will add zest to every effort." It is probably the case that far more pleasure comes from the contriving of means to make a thing "do," and succeeding, than would have resulted from the purchasing of a new one. For the woman who is "dead tired" with planning and contriving, it is doubtless a great relief to buy at once the new thing, but just now, in our country at least, many women are tired for the lack of the pleasure which comes from planning. For planning comes next to creating, and to create is essentially the part of woman.

There would not have been so much pleasure in the Creation if it had not been preceded by chaos. To overcome difficulty is pleasure, because it gives always a sense of power, than which there is nothing more agreeable. To have power, and to use it, is a great joy; just as the possession of power shut out from its exercise is the hardest thing to bear. As to income, then, let us overcome the necessity which confronts us, with our own freedom in invention. Whenever we conquer necessity with freedom, we discover that they are the same, and do not need the dialectic of the metaphysician to convince us of the fact. If we would know of the doctrine, we must do the work; otherwise we shall only humbly trust that it is so.

To secure time for all we have to do, we must offset the rapidity of its flight by reducing as many of our actions as possible to automatism. Doing this,

4

we shall not only perform them more quickly at the time, acting, as we shall, like a machine, but we shall set free a large proportion of the thinking power we have, to be applied to work which may refresh us instead of wearying. I quote from a recent article in the *Andover Review:* "The extension of automatic action in the lower range of faculties is the enlargement of freedom and power in realizing the higher objects of personal life, for it is growing facility in the application of means to ends. The more things a man can do without conscious effort, in the use of his bodily powers, in the use of reasoning faculties, of memory, of languages, of music, the wider range he has in the great pursuits of literature, science, philosophy, art, and religion. He has more power and he has wider area. Animals have more automatic action at the start, but make little appreciable gain upon

it, and get no release for higher uses.
Man, by increasing his unconscious and
subconscious action, of which he has but
little at the start, widens his range continually, and increases the effectiveness
of his personality, which guides native
and acquired powers to the ends he
may choose. And there is no ascer-
tained limit to enlargement of power
through the extension of habitual action into the various facilities of which
man is capable." Leaving aside the
bearing of this fact upon the question
of immortality, of which the writer in
the *Review* goes on to speak, we cannot
read these words without seeing that to
have our thinking power set free from
the common, every-day affairs of daily
life, is exactly the thing we are most
earnestly striving towards. The more
we reduce ourselves to machines in the
lower things, the more force we shall
set free to use in the higher.

When we first began to walk, we had
to give our attention to every step, or
indeed, to the working of every muscle
engaged in taking those steps. We
have only to notice the anxious expres-
sion on the face of the child during his
first lesson in the difficult accomplish-
ment to appreciate this. Now we walk
without thinking of what we are doing.
We can carry on a train of thought while
walking, so deep that we may not know
we are moving at all. This is because
that activity has become automatic. In
psychological language, the lines of discharge of the cells in our brain, necessary to produce in proper order the com-
pound action of walking, have been set
in activity so many times and kept in activity so long at a time, that now all we
have to do is, as it were, to touch off
the explosion of the first cell of the series, and the discharge of the others
follows in regular order. It is like the

fall of a row of card houses. We knock
down the first of the line, and that is
all that is necessary. But if, in our walk,
we come upon an uneven place, we then
at once become conscious of the level
of the ground, and set our foot down
with care; or if it be in a dangerous
spot, with some degree of anxiety. The
course of our thought is checked for
the time, for the thinking power has
had to give its attention to minor matters. When the ground is level again,
the brain hands back the work to its
servants and resumes its own more con-
genial occupation. It is very much the
same with house-keeping. As long
as the house is well organized, and
the daily work running in its habitual
grooves, it runs itself, so to speak. But
if a new emergency arise or a change
of servants occur, the mind of the mis-
tress can no longer be given to her fa-
vorite occupations. She finds herself

dragged down from any thinking on restful themes to the pulverizing cares of daily life until she can reorganize and again deliver over the work to the hands of her executive officers. The multitude of things which we have learned by repeated effort to do automatically is already greater than we should suppose unless we reflect on it, from the very reason that we no longer think about them. Watch the motion of your hands and fingers when buttoning your boot, and you will see how complicated is the seemingly simple act, and how they move with the regularity of the levers in a machine back and forth, back and forth, while you go on talking and have no recollection of having done anything; or, while you are taking a new needleful of thread from the spool as you are sewing, look to see where you are holding your needle. I venture to assert that you do

not know where it has been tucked
away for the moment in order to allow
you the use of your forefinger, and yet
you will find it carefully disposed of, and
by nine hundred and ninety-nine women
out of a thousand in precisely the same
place.   These are good examples of
automatic action.   Did you ever try to
teach any one how to make tatting? If
you have, you will have found out that
although you can do it yourself without
any trouble, you do not really know
how you do it.   The woodsman will tell
in the depth of winter by a glance of
the eye what is the name of the tree,
but he cannot tell you how he knows.
He has so many times observed and
combined in his mind all the characteristics of the tree that he knows it as
soon as he sees it.   To become conscious of processes is the part of a spe-
cialist: it is, for example, to be fit for a
teacher.   In ordinary life, driven as we

modern women are, by so many and differing demands, we must banish all minor matters possible to the region of automatism. And we need not feel that in so doing we are giving up any portion of our prerogative as thinking beings. Just that we might think to some purpose were we gifted with this faculty of performing our work like automata, and in its use lies absolutely our only hope for the present as against the ever-increasing demands of daily life.

We should endeavor to put all things which are of no value in themselves, but are only means to ends, under the control of automatic or mechanical action. There are a hundred things which must be looked after, a hundred orders that must be given, a hundred errands to be done in order that the family may have a comfortable and a restful home. But though they are of importance in that light—for the comfort of other people—they are of no further use. It is important for that day and for that trip that the conductor should have a memory of the faces of the passengers on the train. He goes through the cars many times, and seldom makes a mistake in recognizing a new passenger, or in failing to recognize an old one. This has become automatic with him. But, the trip once over, and the passengers safely disposed of, he clears his memory of them as easily as one washes figures from a slate, and has a fresh memory for the next set as he passes through the train on his next trip, his brain mechanically taking a picture of each car in the train as he goes through for the first time. The girl is going to college. Among the professors under the fire of whose examination she is to come is one who is known to be a great stickler for dates, even to the unit figure, and a warm partisan of a certain authority on ancient dates as opposed to another theory. What is she to do if she is to' pass that examination and gain the privileges of the college? She must commit to memory long lists of dates as important in any culture as the date of the birth of Rameses II. As she has an end to gain she does this, all the time with the consciousness lying back of her mental activity that the list is of no real use to her, further than to reach the Freshman Class. She passes the examination satisfactorily, winning warm commendation from the Professor of History, and in a week's time has forgotten all the dates. This is the story of many an examination and of the knowledge which has been sought in order to pass it. It seems to make a difference in the retaining power of the memory if we know that the facts we are acquiring are to be used

for a special purpose only. What we
learn for the sake of knowing, we hold;
what we learn for the sake of accom-
plishing some ulterior end, we forget so
soon as that end has been gained. This.
too, is automatic action in the constitution of the mind itself, and it is fortu-
nate and merciful that it is so, for otherwise our minds would be soon only
rubbish-rooms.

A very simple and useful device is
to have a memorandum-book, so small
that it can be easily carried in the pocket, to be used instead of your mind to
keep note of any errand or any appoint-
ment that you may have. The Standard Diary, less than four inches long
and less than two and a half inches
wide, is one of the best for this purpose. Besides a page for every day in
the year, it has pages for memoranda,
where you can keep notes of such facts
as the amount of goods needed for any

garment, or trimming for any article
which you are in the habit of using,
so that you will not have to calculate
over and over again the quantity to be
bought. You will not have to stop, as
you are going out, to say, " Let me see !
I forget how much we need of that for
Mary's dress." With true perception of
the value of time, this diary has added
lately a special page for putting down
many of these things, such as number
of gloves, sizes of collar, stockings, cuffs,
shoes, number of bank-book, number of
bicycle, etc. It contains, also, all the
postage rates, directions for help in case
of accidents, antidotes for the most common poisons, the list of divisions for
standard time, church festivals, and all
astronomical information needed, unless by the master of a ship. At the
end is a condensed cash account for
every month of the year, and several
pages devoted to addresses such as

those you are most commonly asked
for and want always at hand : the name
and exact address, for instance, of that
pale - faced young girl who wants sewing to do at home, and whom you want
to recommend to your friends ; that of
the teacher who gave you French lessons last year, and whom you found so
excellent. There are four pages each
given to calls and to letters, with columns for checking them off as returned
or answered. The number of pages allotted to the former would seem to in-
dicate that, in the opinion of the editor
of this diary, it is not likely that a busy
woman will have much time to spend
in making calls which are merely a matter of form, where neither of the parties
engaged can think of anything to say
to the other except at the cost of much
diligent ransacking of the tired brain
and much invention. In fact, such di-
aries as these, in their wide range of

information, would seem to be all that one needs in practical life, the only other book that at all approaches them in this respect being unquestionably Webster's Unabridged Dictionary. And all this information is contained within a tiny well-bound book only half an inch thick, and with excellent paper and type. I speak of the binding because I have repeatedly proved that it will last through the whole year, and be in good order at the end, after having been carried in all sorts of pockets every day and having been opened thousands of times.

As I am speaking of small things, I may be allowed to add that if a rubber ring be put round the first part of the book, shutting up all the past days, it will open always at the place you want, that is, at to-day, so that you will not have to waste any time in hunting for the duties you are in search of. I say

round the first part of the book, because the pages belonging to the coming days want to be left always open
for any engagement you may make for
them. If you have an errand for a certain day, put down the address on the
page where it belongs when you make
the engagement. Then you can dismiss
it from your mind, and when the day
comes you will find it there as you look
over your book for what you have to do
on that day. When you have done the
errand, mark it off then and there by
drawing a line through the memoran-
dum. If at the close of the day you find,
on looking over your artificial memory,
that some of the things have not been
lined off, showing that they have not
been done, transfer these items to the
next page, marking them off with a
cross instead of a straight line. You
will thus be sure that nothing has been
left unthought of, and your work for

each day will, as far as possible, be
shaped out for you in advance. Besides the mental rest which you will
gain by being sure thus that none of all
the little things are forgotten, you will
begin to find an additional amount of
rest, from the feeling which you will
have that your work is laid out for you
—as if you were under the direction of
some one else, and that person one who
is not confused by the multifarious demands of the present, but who plans
for you in quiet and in advance. It is
largely the constant making of decisions
that tires us. To the list of duties for
the day which you find thus prescribed
for you, you will add others as you look
it over in the morning before starting
out on your walk. And when you have
the list complete, arrange your different
errands, if they be many, in the most
convenient order for taking them up,
bearing in mind the street-car routes

and other arrangements of the city
where you live, and jot them down in
order on a card which you can slip under the elastic on the outside of the
book as you drop it into your pocket.
Then follow your list of work laid out
automatically, and you will do your errands with very much less fatigue, being relieved of a hundred little anxieties which, though small, do have a great
cumulative power, and really tire one
more than we should suppose.

If you are a very busy woman, and
must be so, rule the pages of your little
book into columns for morning, afternoon, and evening; or, if it be more
convenient, for in-the-house and out-
of-the-house business respectively, and
you will be still more helped in your
duties for the day by this classification.
I know that some will interpose the ob-
jection here that I am suggesting more
trouble than I shall succeed in avoid-

5

ing. I know well enough that there is
a mania for order in the minds of some
people that really makes more trouble
than the disorder which it seeks to prevent; but I can only say that I am giving the results of the experience of a
very hard-worked woman who has carried on for many years both woman's
and man's work, and that without any
respite, and who yet finds herself now
far stronger and abler for work than
most of the women who have had, compared with her, almost nothing to do.
It can never be often enough repeated
that it is the constant succession of little things and small anxieties that wear
upon us, and not the great things. The
only wise way for us is to hand over as
many little things as possible to the
care of automatism, and to conquer
monotony by bringing larger and more
fruitful interests into our minds in the
space thus left free. It is always a

positive gain of time to make our plans beforehand and in quiet, when we can see clearly. It is like taking directions from Philip sober instead of from Philip drunk, and that saves time and useless work.

As to the smoothness of the house-work, it is an undoubted fact that the reason why so many women have continual trouble with their servants is that they do not give clear directions, and then find fault because the directions are not followed, or they make such uncertain and varying demands that the best and most anxious to please become discouraged. Servants, as well as any one else, like to have something certain to depend upon, and will serve more willingly often, though they have more to do, where they have their work clearly laid out for them, and where they feel perfectly sure that if they follow orders they are not going to be found fault with. I know that all the fault does not lie directly at the door of the employer, but I think we do not perhaps realize how much of it lies there indirectly. It is a strong desire of the human race to fall back into a state of mechanism. There is nothing which the average mind so strongly and so constantly craves as rules and definite statements. Teachers know this, and their one effort during all the school-hours may be said to be to shake the pupils' minds out of the tendency to mechanism, and to force them into a state of self - activity. But with the house-keeper, the question is not how to train immature minds, but how to get the work done decently and in order. The object for her is the quietness, order, and comfort of the house, and the servants are only means to this end; so she may conscientiously allow them to fall into habits of mechanism as to the greater part of their work. Their

daily routine should be laid out for
them for each day of the week, and
trouble and dispute will be saved by
putting it down in writing, and having
the programme fastened up where they
can refer to it. It is a question of saving time and the annoyance which prevents clear action of the mind, and it
makes not much difference how little
the gain may be, if it be only a gain.
Whatever can be saved in this way will
bear fruit a hundred-fold in the comfort
of those who are dearer to us than ourselves, for there is no Calumet or Hecla
mine that pays so large dividends as
Home.

Let there be constant watchfulness
over the stores always kept in the house,
so that no one of them shall ever be suf-
fered to run out. Always order more before the supply comes quite to an end,
and then you will never be driven to
hurry by an unexpected demand coming

at the most inopportune time, for more
of this or that. It is best always to have
a written list of all these regular stores,
and to be sure in this way that they are.
always on hand, not trusting to your
memory; always save your memory by
paper memories, as to all small details.
The greatest order should be insisted
on, not only in the general household, but in all personal belongings.
There can hardly be too much careful
arrangement here.   The old New England saying of "a place for everything
and everything in its place" is in need
of revival by those of us who want time
saved for relief. If we are not the possessors of an instinct for order, we must
create and diligently cultivate it. As
to the many small articles of a woman's
wardrobe —which should always be so
arranged that she can get any of them
in the dark as well as in the light—a
little of the invention, always necessary

if we are to find our way out of the difficulty that we are living in, will be sufficient to instruct a carpenter so that
there may be in the top drawer a place
for everything, out of which it cannot
slip because of partitions which shut it
in. I have a friend who has her shoe-
drawer also arranged in divisions, so
that she never has to stop to hunt for
the mate to a shoe, the pairs lying always together. Some may think this
a useless thing, but I happen to know
that this woman does an almost incredible amount of work in different lines,
and that she never keeps anybody who
has an engagement with her waiting for
one moment. These results may seem
worthy of attainment, as they certainly
enable her to meet the many calls upon
her attention in a quiet frame of mind.
It is the little foxes that spoil the vines,
and the little things that tell upon nervous strength. At the desk, whenever

anything is done with, it should be at
once restored to its place, and not left
lying round to be looked up when wanted again.   Pencils, rulers, and blotters
should come under this stern rule, the
carrying out of which will soon form a
habit, and save in the total a great
amount of time.   These are only the
simplest rules of business. As it is undoubtedly an advantage to American
homes that so many of the wives and
mothers have served as teachers before
becoming house-directors, so it will be
an advantage that so many young wom-
en are getting now some degree of training through their employment in offices
and at cash-desks. They will carry with
them into their future homes the business habits there acquired, which are
only the gradually summed-up experience of many generations of business
men interested in doing things in the
shortest possible time, and the homes

will be benefited thereby. Before you begin to work, see that every one of the small tools you are to use is in the most convenient place for reaching it, so that you may not have to make one unnecessary movement, and you will be surprised to find with how little expenditure of force you will do the work. Few women probably reflect, as they sit in their comfortable chairs at a theatre and enjoy the smooth performance without a hitch or break, upon the amount of order and preparation indispensable to produce the result which charms them. A visit to the property-room and a little talk with the man or woman in charge might be a good lesson upon the effect of thorough order and previous arrangement in preventing friction. You see the actor reach for the pen or for some little thing required by the play, and you do not think that it was the business of some one to see that all these

little unnumbered trifles should be in
the particular place where they were
wanted at precisely the time when they
were wanted; and the next day at din-
ner you find fault sharply with the servant because necessary articles are not
on the table. Perhaps it was not the
fault of the servant so much as that of
some one else. It is little things like
these that destroy the whole comfort of
a dinner-table, and vex and annoy others besides yourself. It is so much easier
to prevent trouble than to cure it! A little more order in the household arrangements, a little more carefully planned
directions to the servants, and, above
all, a little more of the oversight of the
trained eye beforehand, would save so
much friction and spare yourself so
much fatigue; for most of the women
who will read these words are not tired
with bodily labor directly, but only with
the exhaustion coming from the men-

tal friction which follows them every
day, and with the constant effort to
keep things smooth and to do all their
duty.

So closely are the mind and body
related that the very effort at keeping
things in order will tend to spread order
in the thought, so that clear thinking
and clear directions, which are its result, will day by day become easier.
Go on, patiently putting and keeping
outside things in order, and you will
find that after a while you are beginning to gain a mental grip of the problems which beset you. They will fall
into order, and take their places according to their proper relations. It is useless trying to have any real order in a
school of children where the maps on
the walls are awry, chairs and tables
crooked, and the interiors of the desks
a scene of wild confusion, as if the
books had been tipped in like coal from

a cart. So you are not able to think in order clearly and logically in a room where everything is in confusion. In the same way, if you want to rest with your mind, you must learn first of all to keep all parts of the body quiet—that is, to have them under control. If you try to stop a street-car, and the driver takes no notice of you, diligently regarding the fine proportions of a steeple in the distance, though you may not yet be able to see him go by with profound quietness of mind, you can at least refrain from expressing your feelings. After you have done this a sufficient number of times, holding yourself in perfect serenity so far as the outward woman is concerned, you will be agreeably surprised to find that you begin not to be so provoked as was your wont. Try it. Learn not to play with your watch-chain, not to swing your shopping-bag slowly back and forth, not per-

petually to caress the handle of your
umbrella as you ride. Learn to keep
still, and you will feel the quieting influence all through your life. If the
train stops, don't ask a hundred questions, which don't concern you, as to
the cause of the delay. Do not seek
for information of which you can make
no use. When the steamer goes slowly
because of fog, do not attack the cap-
tain every time he appears on deck with
your inquiries as to whether he thinks
he will run into an iceberg or another
vessel, or whether there is always fog
in that part of the ocean, and a hundred others, so various as to leave no
doubt in the mind of any one who lis-
tens to them of the great power of invention of their propounder. The cap-
tain will perhaps answer, gruffly, as I
heard one do, that he has never lived
there and can't tell. The woman who
received this answer felt doubtless that

she had been hardly treated, but she had only herself to blame.

Learn to keep still outwardly, even as to hands and the tips of your fingers, as to feet and head, and you will find rest and quiet coming to the mind as a result. If you are ill, lie quiet if it be possible, and it will generally be found so. Lie still, and don't allow yourself to toss about. Sit still when you sit, and stand still when you must stand. Try this constantly and persistently and you will not fail of help. Allow yourself to make no motion that has not a purpose and an aim; if you find yourself moving unnecessarily, call yourself back to quietness. No one can tell how much of the beautiful serenity of the Quakers comes from the outward stillness and quiet of their worship. Watch other people to be convinced how much muscular and nervous force is actually thrown away for nothing.

Do not allow yourself to move nerv-
ously fast, and the more nervous you
are, the more deliberate all motions
should be.   Force yourself to move
slowly even if you are in a hurry.   In
walking, the tread of the city policeman
is an excellent model for one to imitate,
though there is no danger that you will
succeed in copying it exactly.   When
at your desk and with not much time,
to spare, the pencil falls on the floor,
and the ruler won't be picked up, your
eye-glass string catches on a button,
you can't find the blotter, and the paper on which were the memoranda you
were copying just gets up from the
desk and plunges, without any obvious
motive-power but its own will, into the
waste-basket; or when, another day,
scissors slip to the floor, the knot which
you are sure you had made at the end
of your basting-thread is not there, the
button-hole-twist kinks, knots, and, tak-

ing on a life of its own, becomes a self-
flinging lasso in pursuit of any game,
and the needle, going through perilous-
ly hard, finally snaps into three pieces;
in short when—to use Gail Hamilton's
felicitous phrase—the "total depravity
of inanimate things" is manifestly in
the ascendant, that is the time for delay and dallying. When you are waiting for a train, don't keep perpetually
looking to see if it is coming. The
time of its arrival is the business of
the conductor, not yours. It will not
come any sooner for all your nervous
glances and your impatient pacing, and
you will save strength if you will keep
quiet. After we discover that the people who sit still on a long railroad journey reach that journey's end at precisely the same time as those who
"fuss" continually, we have a valuable
piece of information which we should
not fail to put to practical use.

If you were asked to raise one hundred and twenty pounds twelve or thirteen feet you would probably answer that you were not strong enough to do it; and yet that is what you do every time that you go up a flight of stairs. You do not think of that, but it is worth while for you to do so, and to make wise choice of the muscles with which you will do the work. It is not the best way to place only the ball of your foot on the stair, throw yourself forward, and then do the lifting with the muscles of the back. If, instead of this, you will plant the whole foot on the step, and then simply straighten the knee, keeping yourself perfectly erect, you will find that much fatigue is saved; and in city houses there are many stairs to be climbed in the course of a day. Take care of yourself in such little ways as these. Try in every way to acquire a habit of quietness. God has

6

mercifully built us so that habits are easily formed. Help yourself out of the stores of aid which He has provided for you from the foundation of the world.

And if you must have tonics, take those also from Him, in sunshine, pure air, exercise, regular hours, healthful food, and, above all perhaps, in sleep. Religiously avoid all others. It is vain hoping to restore nerve-power by recourse to medicine. All such attempts are but patches, which only take from the garment, making the rent worse. An English physician has recently said of the maladies which imply or consist in loss of nerve-power, such as suppressed gout, hysteria, neuralgia, insomnia, chorea, epilepsy, melancholia, and general loss of mental control, that " all this class of ills are, as a rule, whether they be hereditary in their origin or not— and very often they are hereditary—ex-

tremely gradual and slow in their onset,
arising, as they do, from deep-rooted,
constitutional causes." He maintains,
therefore, that they can be successfully
combated " only by very cautious and
gradual remedies — remedies which do
not cause any reaction but which slowly steal into the system, and restore
its strength by gradually accumulating,
without stimulating, the resources from
which nerve-power is derived. Strong
nerve-tonics are in such cases mischiev-
ous, and sedatives positively injurious.
A healthy plan of life, with air, exercise,
and nutritive food are of the first importance." This point can hardly be
enough insisted upon. What you have
done by a long series of drafts upon
your nerve strength, whether necessary
or not, can be made up only by a long
series of efforts at patience and of will-
power to keep yourself still and in the
way of recovery. You cannot hurry

the processes of the Creator, however
much you may desire to do so—

"Though the mills of God grind slowly, yet
they grind exceeding small."

If you have learned by experience of
the exceeding smallness of the grinding, you must also learn practically of
the exceeding slowness of the machin-
ery.   There is no other way.

We should hardly go to Earle's *English Prose* to find advice about bodily
health, and yet at the foot of page 210
is this sentence : "Ailing people fancy
that some specific might in a minute
put them all to rights if only they could
chance upon it; not considering that
health is the result of a harmonious condition of a highly complex organization,
and that the main secret lies in the con-
duct and regulation of that life which is
its animating centre."   Professor Earle
is speaking of diction, and of the idea

which many writers have, that "it is a
sovereign specific of diction to use
short words." If the practice of medicine consisted in the giving of specifics,
physicians would be of very little use.
All that we should need would be a
book with the remedy for every trouble
set down in a column opposite to the
name of the disease. Teachers are very
often confronted by the same miscon-
ception on the part of parents, who seem
to think that instruction, instead of being a live process, consists in a sort of
knack, a certain method which has only
to be applied to the children like a plas-
ter, to insure success in the school.
They seem to think that teachers have
in some way been inducted into a secret method, and that anybody could
teach if he were a participator of the
secret "method." This is the idea of
all quackery, in whatever profession,
and the fact that so many who have

over-used their nerve-force expect to re-
cover at once, if only they could find
the tonic suited to their case is a proof
how wide-spread is the belief in quackery and quacks. If you are nerve-tired,
do not be induced to trust to tonics of
any kind, and never to sedatives if you
hope to make any real gain.   Tea, cof-
fee, and alcohol will not help you now.
You have used them before as your al-
lies in evading obedience to the plain-
est rules of health ; do not hope that
they will act as such in the effort to re-
gain it.   And remember always that
you must give some thought, and a considerable amount of it, too, to the care
of your health if you expect to be of
any use in the world, or comfort to anybody.   It is only in such ways as have
been here indicated that you can meet
the demands of modern life, and conquer necessity.   What you are to try
to acquire above all is what the *Satur-*

day Review characterizes as " repose,
and the calm power frequently associ-
ated with it which is greatly lacking in
the sons and daughters of the latter
part of the nineteenth century." Look
carefully through all the claims pressing upon you in your complicated life,
and decide once and for all what it is
that is the one really important and
overmastering duty in it, and should
be the one dominating aim. Then remember that if you succeed in that, the
others, so multifarious, are really no
more than the fringe of the garment,
and that you need not spend so much
anxiety over them, provided that the one
most important is faithfully attended to.
What that is for each woman, no other
person can decide for her.

III

FREEDOM

ALL real freedom springs from necessity, for it can be gained only through the exercise of the individual will, and that will can be roused to energetic action only by the force of necessity acting upon it from the outside to spur it to effort. The necessity, as we call it, under which we labor, comes mostly from the outside and from the physical world, while the freedom to which it leads or rather pushes us is of the spirit. There is no real contradiction between the two. Our "must" is determined by the direction in which we voluntarily set our faces, and so is superimposed upon us

by our own wills.   We set up a certain
aim, and put ourselves of our own will
into the power of a certain current.
Once having done that, we find ourselves committed to usages and customs
which we had not before fully known,
but from which we cannot depart without giving up the end which we have
chosen.   But we have no right, therefore, to claim that we are under the
yoke of necessity.   We might as well
say that the man whom we see struggling
vainly in the current of Niagara could
not have helped jumping in.   He de-
liberately chose the leap and preferred
to trust himself to the water rather than
to the land, and he was allowed his
choice.   The woman who marries because she desires diamonds and foreign
travel, and gets both, has no right to
complain afterwards that she has no
love or companionship, and no home.
She made her bargain, and was paid in

the coin that she asked, and fully. She
chose her own lot, and should accept
it in silence and not talk about "hard
fate." The woman who makes her en-
trance into a set of society must not
complain if she finds that society is
satisfied with no half-hearted devotion.
She has lost the right to say that she
has no time for such or such a duty.
She has all the time that there is, all
that any one can have; she has chosen
to spend it in a special direction; it is
not that she has not had it to apply as
she chose.

The feverish emulation of Americans
to excel each other in the ways of "society" is responsible for a large amount
of the weariness and the nervous pros-
tration which are charged-up against
necessary demands upon our time,
though they do not belong there. Maria
Mitchell used to say to women who,
pleading for help, urged that they "must

live,'' that there was not the slightest
necessity for living, and, moreover, that
if there were, the almshouse was always
open, a fact which she declared to be
of great comfort to herself. It was only
her brusque way of saying that many
things which people generally put in
the domain of the necessary really do
lie in that of the unnecessary, or of
freedom. Those women who read *Mar-
cus Aurelius*, and who know that "the
life is more than meat and the body
than raiment," do not need to be told
where Freedom lies. The others who
cry piteously for more freedom may
have come across the statement, "Who
would be free, themselves must strike
the blow," but have perchance never
thought that it referred to any one but
the Swiss mountaineers or the struggling
patriots of Greece. To be free in any
sense, a certain amount of independence
is necessary, nor can Freedom be pur-

chased at any other price.   It would
seem imperative that society, so called,
should exist, for otherwise how would
the horses have their manes pulled and
their tails docked, each one blunter
than the other ; and what would become
of the manufacturers of bearing-reins ?
There must be a gilded image to set up
if we are going to build a temple.   These
facts seem irrefragable.   But there is one
thing sure : the carpenter who does not
believe in Unions, and who keeps out
of them as long as possible, only to join
at last, and never afterwards dares to
express his honest opinion, or his sense
of justice, is no more an absolute slave
than is the woman who surrenders her
own action, in whatever direction, to the
dictates of society.   Both she and the
carpenter are under a slavery as absolute as if they were living in Russia or
Turkey, and they will not come out until
they have paid the uttermost farthing.

Many women seem to be under the
impression that nothing can be accomplished in the direction of freedom unless a Society be formed with president,
vice-president, secretary, treasurer, and
a large board of directors, and public.
meetings held. But independence does
not lie that way. There are many things
that perhaps you would like to do or
like to have; first bear in mind the undoubted truth that there are perhaps
only one or two things in the world
which are not far more charming in desire than they are in possession. Montaigne relates how ardently from his
earliest youth he had desired to have
the order of St. Michael conferred upon
him. But when he had in his hand the
coveted decoration, it had ceased to attract him, partly because through his
growth he no longer held it in so high
esteem, partly also, probably, because it
was his. The great actor who at last

realized the dream of his life in owning a theatre is said to have had no pleasure in it when he had built it and could fill it night after night with a delighted public. For pleasure lies in pursuit, not in the attainment. It is because of this, that society is never satisfied, and, however wearied, is always on the race-track, straining every nerve to reach the goal.

But where we cannot acquire all things, we must have some measure of values in order to select. That measure will be the one great aim of our lives, whatever it may be. If we have no aim, then of course we have no measure ; and in that case it does not matter to ourselves or to any one else that we have none, so we may be left out of the account. The Rev. Edward E. Hale, in one of his fictitious - real stories, describes the experiment of shooting a train of cars across the abyss

round which the Horseshoe Bend runs
. on the Pennsylvania Railroad, in order
to save time, and he details with Swift-
like minuteness the abstruse mathemat-
ical calculations as to rate of speed and
precise point of projection.   He then
goes on to describe the actual trying of
the experiment and its gratifying success.   The train, he tells us, landed
safely on the other side at the very
point calculated, with the exception of
the drawing-room car, which, being last
and becoming detached, had fallen into
the gulf.   But he says this in no wise
detracted from the complete success,
because passengers who travel in drawing-room cars would never be missed
by any one, and that therefore they
and their fate may with propriety be
dropped altogether from the results,
like infinitesimal quantities in a mathe-
matical calculation.   The humor is de-
licious, and may serve to hint at a truth.

At least those who have no particular aim in life really are of no account; their various actions are as likely as not to cancel each other, and whatsoever happens to them can never furnish material for a tragedy. But a fixed aim furnishes us with a fixed measure, by which we can decide whether such or such an action proposed is worth trying for or not, and as aims must vary with the individual, the decisions of any two people as to the desirableness of an action may not be the same. But a certain proud independence you must possess if you would have peace of mind.

Commenting on the suicide of a prominent banker, the Boston *Transcript* says: "Let us get rich as fast as we can. Let us speculate. Let us make fortunes and lose them, maybe; no matter about that—but make them, anyway. Let us cut ourselves off from the sweet and wholesome influences of life,

and give ourselves up to fever and mad-
ness. Never mind about the conse-
'quences to our own peace of mind of
such a course. Our own peace of mind
is never worth considering. Can you
put up peace of mind with a bank as
collateral for a loan? Will the Street
reckon your peace of mind among your
assets? Why, no; and what the Street
does not value, is worthless, of course.
And yet many a man dies for want of
this very thing." The words are too
sadly true. Yet peace of mind is an
undoubted security at a high rate of
interest. It is unavailable as collateral
only because it is non-negotiable—nobody can transfer title to peace of mind;
but its value is not thereby affected,
since nobody ever desires to pledge or
exchange it for anything. It is your
business to find the bank that deals
in it.

Advice has been defined to be "that
7

which everybody wants, everybody asks
for, everybody gives, and nobody takes."
But certainly there is a lack of truth in
the last assertion. The rider buys a
horse which is perfect in every way
and suits him exactly. But a friend
suggests that it is not quite up to his
weight, another remarks that it is a little nervous, and a third finds some fault
with the shape of a spot on the nigh
fore-leg. All these criticisms work si-
lently in his mind after the way of unconscious cerebration, and three weeks
after we meet him riding another animal. He has simply taken advice;
that is all. How many of the books
that you have read during the last year
have you read simply and only because
some one said, "You really ought to
read it!" How many changes in your
dress have you made on account of the
half-meant criticism of a friend. How
much trouble might you not have saved

if, instead of consulting with another as
to some annoyance, you had only sat
down in your own room—if your closet
seemed to you too small — applied to
the difficulty the measure of your life,
and quietly decided your course of action for yourself. The truth is that too
much, not too little, is taken of the un-
thinking advice tossed at us every day,
often forgotten by the giver. We need
to preach the gospel of independence
in America, not that of dependence.
We are always going, as we think,
with the majority. But we forget that
the greater majority is an invisible one,
and that it may be safer to side with
that. It is not alone individuals that
take too much advice. Our Legislat-
ures and even Congress — it may be a
result of the peculiar manner of electing
their members—often yield, as in utter
helplessness, on the most important is-
sues, to advice, no matter whence com-

ing. A society of women, well-meaning, but with thought totally possessed by one evil, that of drunkenness, asks permission to offer advice to the Legislature. The legislators thereupon frame a law, requiring all text-books in physiology which are to be used in the public-schools to be profusely illustrated with violent wood-cuts, depicting the liver or the stomach of an habitual drinker, and a chapter to be attached to every division of the book, pointing out the effect of alcohol on the different tissues of the body. They think to produce in the child's mind a terror of the distantly possible which will enable the man to turn away from the saloon. If they were teachers, they would place a more just estimate on the residuum left in the minds of children from such talk in school. Or Congress obediently follows the advice of the manufacturers of some article and lays a high duty upon

it, only to wake to the knowledge, a few
months later, that in protecting that
infant industry they have throttled in
a distant territory half a dozen others,
of whose indirect connection with the
first, they had never had even the shade
of the shadow of an idea. Mr. Powder-
ly would not probably materially im-
prove the Constitution were it to be
subjected to his revision, as was seri-
ously proposed only a few years ago.
Everybody takes advice, because it
seems to be a way of getting, at least
temporarily, out of a difficulty, and, at
any rate, of shifting the responsibility
for failure if it come.   But the fact is
that there is only one person who can
decide a problem, because he is the
only one knowing all the conditions,
external and internal, and that is the
person whose problem it is.   You have
to grapple with it first or last, and it is
as easy to do it first.   Free yourself at

once from the slavery of always doing this or that just because some friend says to you, "You really ought to do it!" and you will take the first step towards an independence which will rest you, if it be only on account of its novelty. In a recent article in the *Fortnightly Review*, entitled "Under the Yoke of the Butterflies," Mr. Auberon Herbert says: "The world persistently presents us with the paradox that a very large percentage of its people live habitually doing what they don't want to do: giving subscriptions they don't want to give; visiting and receiving people they don't want to visit and receive; saying things they don't mean and don't want to say; spending time and money which they don't want to spend; supporting measures and proceedings they don't want to support; putting into this or that kind of office people whom they would rather not see there; in fact, generally contradicting themselves, because they have attached themselves to some system or other which they find it is, on the whole, easier to obey than to disobey."

In the matter of dress it seems as if the majority of women have no independence at all. If, as has been said, every woman creates in her own likeness the gifts which are given her, it is surely true that every woman should in a measure create after her own nature the dress which she habitually wears. To see two grown women dressed exactly alike is, with almost every one, to pass the mental judgment that at least one of them must have very little character of her own. In a somewhat restricted sense we pass the same judgment when each season we see almost every woman in a city following some one decree of fashion, no matter how unreasonable, inconvenient, or unbecoming. Fash-

ion says, " Fasten your arms down to
your hips so that you will look like a
trussed turkey," and they do it. " Have
your sleeves set up so that it will be impossible to lift your hands to your
heads, so that you will have to put on
your hat before you put on your dress,"
and the obedient slaves answer, " Aye."
" Sweep the streets with your skirts,"
and they are swept. " Wear them so
tightly drawn that the outline of your
form is distinctly seen by every one
who may meet you," and a life school
for the sculptor is at once set up in every street-car. These illustrations are
perhaps enough, though the list might
be almost indefinitely enlarged. It is
by no means to be maintained that fashion has not a certain right to authority.
As Walter Pater acutely says, " The
power of fashion is but one minor form,
slight though it may be, yet distinctly
symptomatic of that deeper yearning

of human nature towards an ideal perfection which is a continuous force in
it." To ignore fashion entirely, or to
fight against it continually, is not to secure freedom. It is said that one of
the sweetest and strongest of Boston
women, now dead, but while here always anxious to serve others, made herself more trouble and care by insisting
upon the really uncouth dress which
she habitually wore than if she had con-
formed to the prevailing style, simply
because her attire was so out of date
that it was hard and almost impossible
to have it made after her plans. It is
not necessary to go to such extremes
as this. It is perfectly easy for any
woman so to dress that, while she is not
noticeable on the street, she shall be
entirely comfortable, and able to do
what she has to do without fatigue
from carrying undue weight, and without having any motion consciously ham-

pered. I heard one woman say to another some years ago: "Oh, do get a Jersey waist. You have no idea how comfortable they are! Why, I can lift both arms up straight over my head." And she did so, stretching up her shapely arms with a sigh of relief and a smile of triumph, only to hear the answer, "Why, I have not a dress in the world that I cannot do that in. And the speaker, too, lifted her arms, straight as an arrow high above her head, while all the weight of her skirts was lifted smoothly and easily, as the shoulders rose. And yet you would not have remarked the dress of the second woman if you had met her, as at all peculiar. It is not necessary, in order to reform your dress, if it need reforming, to belong to any association or any league for the purpose. As the most natural and effective way after the war to resume specie payments was just simply

to resume, so the most sensible way to
reform your dress is to reform it. Any
woman whose dress is worth considering at all, surely has enough common-
sense and invention to order her own
under-clothing so that it shall be healthful and perfectly comfortable. If she
have not, she had better not try to reform the world in any larger way. There
is one thing sure : if you will not trouble yourself much about the passing
fashion, taking care only not to dress
so that you will attract attention from
excessive singularity, but keeping all
the parts of your clothing simple and
comfortable, you will be sure to see the
fashion come round to you once in
about seven years, and find yourself, to
your great amusement, wearing clothes
in the mode. The original Free Soil-
ers were a small party at first but it
took only time for all the Whigs to fall
into line after them.

At any rate, if you are to do your work without getting tired, you have got to save all unnecessary weight in what you have to carry, and what weight cannot be avoided should be hung where it will do the least harm. The amount of strength which can be saved by conforming to the simplest rules of common-sense in the matter of dress is very great, as those of us who have tried it know. Of course the object of the dress-maker and the tailor is to avoid wrinkles, and they are right, so far as their profession goes; but I fancy you would hardly care to assert that your object in life was the same. It is only the old story; first make up your mind what you want to do with your life, and then decide the question of dress, as every other question, by that test. It is not so hard as you suppose to be independent about these things. Those who are single-hearted in any

great aim never find it so. In fact,
they don't think about it at all. They
go on and do what they have to do,
saving every smallest bit of strength as
they go, and that is all there is about it.

The same necessity of independence
exists as to what you shall read. Most
people read every year what happens
to come in their way, or what some person happens to say that they ought to
read. Just look back over your reading for the last year and say if this has
not been so with you. If you read stories for rest and relaxation, take only
those that are by authors of some real
repute. Eschew the crowd of novels
that every week brings forth, only to
be relegated in a few weeks to de-
served oblivion. Better wait a while,
and see whether a book has any but an
ephemeral life before you spend your
time on it; it is not necessary that you
should read a story at the same time

with everybody else. Do not destroy all the fibre of your mind and lower your whole mental tone by reading wishy-washy stuff, even though it be not bad. And even with the magazines, which give you a series of disconnected articles, inviting you monthly or weekly to an exhibition of noses, arms, hands, and chippings from many studios, but not one really whole work of art, have some line in your reading. As it does not become your duty to visit a woman simply because she invites you to do so, so it is by no means your duty to read an article merely because the editor of a certain magazine serves it up to you. You do not feel obliged to eat of every dish on the bill of fare at a hotel, or to buy all the jewelry in a store because you go into it. The editor makes up his magazine to suit all tastes " if by any means he may please some." If he be worthy of his title,

whether he be magazine or newspaper,
editor, he tries to place himself behind
the public and to see through their eyes.
He endeavors to make each number of
his production a whole in itself, minis-
tering to each of his world of readers in
some way.   In this effort at wholeness
in each number lies the pleasure of his
labor, and in the success of this effort
consists his right to his title.   But that
is no reason why you should read all
he offers.   Read no article in a magazine which does not bear on your own
subjects of thought and does not fall
into line with your other reading, and you
will be doing wisely.   The trouble with
magazines is the same as with concerts :
they consist of only fragments.   If one
of these is such as you need to fill in a
gap in your thought, then you want it.
Pick it out and fit it into your mosaic.
But if you are desirous of understand-
ing Wagner in the degree possible to

you, it would seem hardly worth while to listen to a dozen " Prize Waltzes " before the music of Tannhäuser is played. At the concert you may be obliged to hear many such waltzes in order to reach your aim, but with the magazine the same trouble does not exist. Have always some reason for reading a magazine article or let it alone. The same rule should apply to the daily newspaper. History in the making is a very uncertain thing. It might be better to wait till the South American republic has got through with its twenty-fifth revolution before reading much about it. When it is over, some one whose business it is, will be sure to give you in a digested form all that it concerns you to know, and save you trouble, confusion, and time. If you will follow this plan, you will be surprised to find how new and fresh your interest in what you read will become. The difference be-

tween reading to find out something
you really want to know, and reading
whatever happens to fall into your hands
is very great. It is like the difference
between eating because you are hungry,
and eating because you are summoned
to the table.

And one word more on the subject
of reading : If you read only the best,
you will have no need of reading the
other books, because the latter are
nothing but a rehash of the best and
the oldest. To read Shakespeare, Pla-
to, Dante, Milton, Spenser, Chaucer,
and their compeers in prose, is to read
in condensed form what all others have
diluted. If you have little time for eating, you will find it desirable to take
only the most nutritious food—that is,
only the most condensed. Do the same
thing as to books, and you will be surprised to find how much time you will
have for reading.

8

Then how much strength and time
do you waste every day in worrying
about possible happenings, half of which
never come to pass? With a little reasoning and a little determined effort of
will, there is a chance for great economy
in this line. When your friend is ill, you
suffer a hundred deaths for one which
perhaps will not come, because you give
rein to your excited imagination, and
arrange in your mind for all sorts of
future contingencies. If instead of doing this you will give your whole attention to the actual present, doing faithfully all that can be done, and then just
leave something to God, you will save
so much wear and tear. Many people
are not willing to leave anything entirely in His hands, and practically treat
Him as if He were far from as com-
petent as themselves. It is precisely
"in all time of our tribulation" that we
should trust the most. One is often

reminded of the little boy who was quite willing to say his prayers at night, but absolutely refused to say them in the morning, maintaining that "any fellow could take care of himself in the day-time." And yet those who will not practise trusting in the sunshine are sure to find difficulty in the darkness. We cannot expect to reap where we have not sown, though we often for that reason

> "all alone beweep our outcast state,
> And trouble deaf Heaven with our bootless
> cries."

There was much wisdom in the story in the old reading-books of the farmer's clock, which stopped one night because the pendulum had been calculating how many times it would have to beat in a century, and felt itself entirely discour-aged at what was to be required of it. But the centuries are not dealt out to us in wholes. We persist in winding up our eight-day clocks every evening, and then wonder that we are so tired. We laugh at Don Quixote as he tilts with windmills, and then close the book to do the same thing. It is not impossible to control imagination. It may be hard; but fighting, even if it bring temporary defeat, is better than not fighting, and what seems defeat is often victory, even if we do not count the increased strength which comes from effort of the will. The farmers had to retreat from Bunker Hill, but they won a victory all the same. It was for us that those ten thousand kinsmen of ours stood against the hosts of the Persians at Marathon, and won the fight because of the invisible forces within them. They are fighting for us still, and we with them, if we fight at all. And then

The sun *will* shine and the clouds will lift;
The snow will melt, though high it drift;
Across the ocean there is a shore;
Must we learn the lesson o'er and o'er?

To know there is sun when the clouds droop
  low,
To believe in the violets under the snow,
To watch on the bows for the land that shall
  rise—
That is victory in disguise.

There can be no work, whatever it
may be, that is so exhausting as pain-
ful emotion ; while on the other hand,
mercifully, there is no tonic so upbuild-
ing and renewing as joy, which sets into
active exercise every constructive power of the body, and whose rush is like
the leap of the brooks in spring from
the strong mountain-tops to the low-
lands. There is nothing more sure to
undermine health than constant gnaw-
ing dissatisfaction with one's lot. And
that is in your own power to destroy,
though you may not be able to alter
the circumstances. Emily Dickinson
said a wise thing when she wrote, "Do
not try to be saved, but let redemption
find you, as it certainly will." She might
have added, as she surely meant, if you

keep in the roads by which it travels.
In most cases of nervous exhaustion it
is the diseased mind which requires
treatment, or has required treatment
long before. "Useless muscular tension is merely a reflex of cerebral conditions." The body is only the tool of
the mind, and its restlessness betrays
the condition of that mind. Do not
waste much time by treating symptoms;
if you want to be cured, go straight to
the cause of the disease. Medical science will tell you that more and more
it relies for a cure on the great healing
forces of Nature. If the physician can
succeed in giving strength to the tone
of the whole body, he knows that he may
leave the disease to take care of itself.
Only a temporary peace is gained by a
treaty which does not touch the under-
lying principles that caused the war.
And there will always be restlessness
and fatigue till peace is born of inner
freedom.

IV

RESTLESSNESS

HE migration of whole races from their original homes, in the history of the world generally westward to new locations, has been a phe- nomenon always especially interesting to the student of history, considering not only the great changes which it has involved in the lives of the nations upon which they have poured down, but also the causes that have induced the movement. It seems as if a whole people becomes possessed by a kind of fury for a change. They leave all that is familiar to them and go in a mass to strange places, driving out be- fore them the inhabitants of those lands

and taking the country for their own.
Why they should do so at that time
more than at any other is to us inscruta-
ble, except that, in the Scripture phrase,
"the fulness of time" is come for them.
History is full of such stories, from the
great irruption of the Mongol Tartars
into China to the risings and departures
of the peoples in the north of Europe,
whose far-off rush southward made itself at last very distinctly felt in the
fall of the Roman Empire, and that also
when the "fulness of time" was come.
When Christianity turned the main
forces of the world inward, it did not
leave untouched this impulse for movement. The area to be sought and taken
possession of was, in a measure, trans-
ferred to the spirit, and the restlessness
which had long before driven those old
tribes to wide wandering now appears in
the mind instead of on the surface of
the earth. The wandering goes on still,

and in mighty hordes of men, over wide
and unknown spaces. The old land-
marks are forsaken, and a strong impulse, not confined to any one country
or continent, calls thought forth to new
and untried conquests. The old impulse is not dead; only its field has
been changed. The migration is now
into the fields of natural science, now
into those of divine truth, and it presses
always further. Old standards are cast
aside, old conceptions put to the test;
the demand is for change, always change,
and for new resting-places for thought
and belief. The human spirit is always
asking after a place where it may stop
and build abodes. But so long as it is
human—which is the same thing as divine—it must be driven, in spite of its
own will, by the impulse to move on to
new homes. The fever of migration is
contained within its very nature, and it
can hope to escape it only for a time.

To us, who live so close to the twentieth century, the on-rushing movement which sweeps the world away seems to have been accelerated with frightful velocity within the present generation. It seems as if our parents, or at least our grandparents, dwelt quietly among their own folk, and were allowed quietly to die in the old beliefs which they had learned at the knees of their mothers. But for us there is no such repose of soul.

> "'For you,' they said, 'no barriers be,
> For you no sluggard rest.
> Each street leads downward to the sea,
> Or landward to the West.'"

It is possible that we mistake, and that what at this distance appears to us a halcyon rest was to them a time of heart-searching; to them also it may have seemed as if all moorings were loosening, and they drifting with their generation to unknown seas. But, however this may be, we know that for us

the world of invention and discovery
has moved faster than our power to
adapt ourselves to it has increased, and
we, desirous as we are at tired mo-
ments of something that we can rest in,
are forced to consider problems which
in our ignorance we had fancied long
ago settled, so differently do they present themselves to modern thought.
Always there is something new, and
life heaves with a perpetual restlessness, from the influence of which no
one can hold himself entirely free.

It seems to some of us as if what
was known as the old home-life were
fast disappearing; young people no
longer seek their pleasures in the home,
but outside of it, and the pleasures are
no longer quiet. This is not their fault.
We may consider it their misfortune;
but, after all, it is a fact that has to be
faced and cannot be overlooked. It is
an unmistakable truth that the family

tie is not so strong as it was a hundred years ago, and that the individuality of the members of a household has to be taken more into account than was formerly the case. Some of the far-reaching effects of the tendency we may deplore, but we cannot avoid; we have to take the world as we find it, and do the best with it as it is. It is true that this doctrine, carried to the uttermost, would have kept Columbus on the other side of the Atlantic, and left electricity to dash about uncontrolled in the atmosphere instead of obeying our command. In some places we might feel it a duty to inculcate the need of change and of faster progress, but the modern American city is certainly not one of these, and there would seem little danger within its walls of laying too much emphasis on the beauty of repose. And, at any rate, even a clergyman cannot be expected to preach both

faith and works on the same Sunday;
if his text be faith, he must teach faith
to the best of his ability, leaving for
that Sunday at least, the great value of
works out of consideration. In like
manner here and now our text is not
motion but Rest.

Whatever other people in other times
have needed, we in America are not
likely to suffer from stagnation, and a
lack of effort to do a hundred things
at a time; what we need are lessons in
rest and repose, and not more of the
restlessness which already runs riot in
every drop of our blood. We cannot
keep still, though we long to do so, and
though increasing weariness warns us
that we are going on towards a break-
down. The restlessness of the sea is
as nothing compared with the restlessness of the American people. At any
rate, in the sea every drop is trying
to get below every other, and thus to

come nearer to one fixed and stable point; but here every drop in the social ocean is, on the other hand, endeavoring to get above every other in some particular, and there is no fixed point at all.

The restless drive of the impulse is creating a new variety of men and women, to be recognized wherever met — and where, over all the surface of the earth, are they not sure to be met? The mental unrest is passing into the physique. How many women do you know who can sit perfectly still or stand perfectly motionless? With how many do you talk who will allow you to finish a sentence without interrupting? How many have the grace of only walking quietly, or of speaking slowly and placidly so that it is a delight to listen? How many whose eyes are not constantly roving? How many who are not always in a hurry, and complaining that everything

always comes at the same time with everything else? To how many houses—
so-called homes—can you go as into a
haven of rest, where everything breathes
quietness and repose? How many men
can even cross the ferry from New York
to Brooklyn without reading vigorously
every one of the few minutes of the
transit, and then crowding to jump off
the boat before she is made fast, with
one eye still on the open newspaper?
How many can quietly let one street-
car go past without running to catch
it, though there are six others behind
within a quarter of a mile? How many
can wait for a train without reading a
few lines in every one of the newspapers
laid out on the news-stand or carefully examining all the colored cartoons
tacked up on the wall?

When you have answered these questions you will begin to appreciate what
a continual hurry most people live in,

and perhaps you may begin to notice how many unnecessary and perfectly objectless motions you yourself are helping to wear yourself out with. There used to be a simple game played with children, in the old times, which it might be worth while to revive : After our elders had answered what seemed to them a sufficient number of ridiculous questions and were tired of our childish fun, they used to set us in a line and propose that we and they should fold our arms, shut our eyes, and see how long we could keep still, and the one who could keep perfectly still the longest was to be called "the best fellow." Perhaps it may have been so, for "composure is often the highest result of power." If only we were restive instead of restless, it would be well for us.

It is undoubtedly true that our climate has much to do with the state of the case. It is impossible for Englishmen to believe many facts which have always been familiar to us; as, for instance, that one can light the gas on a cold winter day by touching the burner with a knuckle, or that sparks may fly from the hair when brushed under the same circumstances. The editor of the *London Journal of Education* professed entire incredulity as to these things when they were told to him a few years ago. To live in such an electrical climate is to be a very different person from those who do not. It is doubtless true that we do live in a "nervous tension produced by climate and habit of hurried life—a tension visible in the astonishing frequency of sudden deaths from overwork and emotion, and an intense fear of opinion, which, so to speak, causes self-love, the sense of personal dignity, to remain permanently raw." So comments the *Spectator*, reviewing an article entitled "The Brand of Cain,"

9

in the *Fortnightly*, charging the people of the United States with readiness to commit and to condone murder. I am inclined to think that the "habit of hurried life" and the sensitiveness to opinion spoken of as morbid states are not co-ordinate causes with, but results of, the climate, the effect of which goes very deep in all the life of this people. But, as I have said, we have to take the world as we find it, and our climate is one of the factors which must not be left out of the problem we have to solve for ourselves and for our children.

Much of the Restlessness we see and feel comes from over-exertion. It is as if the machine had got to working at such a strain that even if we wished we could not stop it. We seem to have become slaves to the blind force of inertia, and our will is no longer of any avail. There is no bichloride of gold treatment for this state, nor is any necessary, for as it is a result not of deficiency of will, but of its abounding strength—a strength born of constant exercise—we have in our own hands the means for our cure. We have strength of will sufficient to force ourselves not to be outwardly restless when we are awake, if only we will use it. It is the people of most will who are in most danger of wearing out, because they have all their lives forced up the unwilling and protesting bodily powers to tasks which were too great for them, as the horse is forced up to the leap which his reason tells him is dangerously high, by the whip and spur of his rider. When we are awake, I said—and, unhappily, if we have habitually overworked our nervous force, we are awake too often when we know that we ought to be asleep. We hear the clock strike, and calculate the number of hours left to us before the time at which the work

of another day must begin, with a sort
of despair, and with an anathema on
the city congregation so heathenishly
thoughtless of the comfort of people
forced to live within sound of their
much-loved clock that they allow the
perfectly useless time-announcer to dis-
turb and trouble them. They themselves live far away from the steeple, so
that they are not disturbed. Only six
hours left, and then presently only five
and then only four! If that clock would
only stop reiterating its dreadful tale of
truth! You remember the Sibylline
leaves and all the stories of Edgar Poe
that you have ever read, and try to
think of something else, or to be chari-
table to the worshippers who own the
clock, but it is all of no use, and the
next day draws pitilessly nearer and
nearer. You can almost hear the sure,
smooth turning of the earth around its
axis, and you wish that Edison would

turn his attention to the problem of adding to the force of friction in that region. And then you remember that the axis is imaginary only, and that even Edison would be of no use, and the Christian clock strikes again!

The fact is only that the vapor will not go back into the casket, the flying horse on which you have insisted on making your journeys will not descend because the wooden peg in his neck has become fast, the mill which was so useful to grind your corn will not stop grinding even in the night-season. These things are your masters now, not your slaves, and the demon of sleeplessness, more horrible and more fatal than the Old Man of the Sea, is upon you, insisting upon your working without, nay, against your will, just as the screw of a vessel whirls round as the wave lifts it out of the water, and shakes her from stem to stern, uselessly and harmfully, as if driven by some demonic power. The demonic power in you, however, is not demonic, but only a heavenly power perverted, just as all the faults of a child are only unregulated virtues. It is nothing but your own will which has become so strong that you are afraid of it. Do not complain, then, nor hesitate to use your will to keep yourself perfectly quiet at any rate. You can if you only think you can. Be greatly thankful that you have the will, and if the clock be heard again, eat something, which by this time you should have learned to have always within reach, it matters not much what. The physiological trouble is that you have too much blood in your brain, and if you can divert a little of this to the stomach to do work there, you may succeed in sleep suddenly. If you are accustomed to lie awake for hours, you had better make a practice of eating before going to bed, preferably some-

thing warm. While you are waiting for
sleep to come to you, you will certainly
be thinking, probably of the very things
which you are most tired of considering; here too, you must use your will to
determine the course of your thought,
and if it persistently goes back to the
avoided topic, you must just as persistently call it away and set it on another
track. What that track shall be matters
not much, but it must be of your own
choosing. As it is by the will that you
have sinned, so it is only by the road of
the will that you can obtain remission
of the penalties you have brought upon
yourself.

To repeat poetry which you know
perfectly, or to count, is not sufficient.
It must be something which involves
some effort of the memory, a list of
incidents which you recall with a little
difficulty, either in your own life or in
the life of some one else, which have a

certain order in regard to time or an arbitrary succession which you have given to them; there must always be some call upon the memory in order to produce the best result. If you make a mistake in .the order of your events, start at the beginning and go through them again, and if you do this over and over, you will soon find that you begin to do it sleepily, and then the battle is won.   Or start at one corner of a room with which you are perfectly familiar, and travel round it, recalling as you go every piece of furniture in its place, with all the small articles which may lie on it, or beneath it, and if you make a mistake, go back to the same · corner, and do not be satisfied till you have gone quite round the room.   This is a very good plan.   Or if you know the position of the letters on the Hammond type-writer, imagine that you have a Remington instead, and try to write on that and spell your words. This device will present a most decided blank before your mental sight, and that is exactly what you want. It is precisely because your mind is not blank that you can't go to sleep. It is said that Kant used to tell his students to "think the wall," and then when they had succeeded in doing that, to "think their thought of the wall." That is also a very good exercise sleepward. The plans which I have suggested above may seem to conflict with the directions of the philosopher, inasmuch as they lead towards the concrete and his towards the abstract; but that makes no difference. They both lead towards a state of muddiness in the mind, and when thought ceases to be clear you may hope it will stop altogether. It may do to rehearse an imaginary sermon to be preached in Trinity church in case you should ever be summoned to officiate there.   You can arrange the heads, and the more you have, the better.   It would be well to begin as an old preacher in Boston is said to have been fond of doing, " Dear brethren, I shall divide my thoughts on this text into four heads, and each of these I shall subdivide into twenty-five minor divisions." That would be an excellent way of starting in.   Sermons of this sort have such soporific power that they have actually been known to affect the members of the congregation who only listened to them.

One thing you must not do, and that is to become deeply interested in the welfare of the imaginary audience, for if you do, you will step into the domain of the emotions, and there is no sleep there ; keep in the line of pure reason and argument.   Never allow yourself to plan what you are to *do ;* don't get into the realm of real action unless it

be past action, and, again and again, be
sure that you make demand on abstract
memory. Then help the process by
lying in such a way as to leave every
muscle in a state of relaxation. In
other words, lie as if you were dead.
Let go of your muscles! You will find
it possible to withdraw your will from
even the tips of the fingers if you make
the effort to do so. Gradually take it
away from every muscle, beginning with
those of the fingers. When they lie
perfectly limp, call in the will from the
arm muscles, one arm at a time, and so
on. You must give close attention to
this withdrawal of the will, and that is
also good, for then you will cease thinking about yourself or any business.
Put yourself as much as possible into
the state of a man who is dead drunk.
You know how expressionless his hands
look? Don't put yours into any definite position; lift them slowly, and then

let them drop where and how they will, and lie as they fall. It may be added that the slow swinging of a hammock is certainly provocative of sleep. There seems to be a direct *drowsying* influence on the brain, produced by the rhythmical swing which gradually grows slower, and finally dies out by imperceptible gradations; and I think that whoever has had a hammock slung in his room will have come to the conclusion that the instinct of the human race was right when it fashioned rockers for the baby's cradle.

It is as much your duty to go to sleep as it is to eat your food. It is your *fault* that you do not, if you will not use every means in your power towards that end. As God meant that you should die, because only in that way could your life come to perfection, so he meant you to sleep while you lived, and to sleep enough to keep you fresh for work,

which also He mercifully ordained as a
means of health. Just as you withdraw
from the company of friends and un-
dress yourself, so you should take your
mind to itself, free it from the gar-
ments necessary to labor, and put it
into His hands for refreshment and
rest. But you do not do this when you
lie down only to go over and over the
actions of the finished day, or painfully
to lay plans for the cares of the morrow. .It is especially futile to try to do
this last ; what you will do when the day
comes must depend very much upon
what sort of a day it is, and what shall
be the conditions of the real work-a-day
world. Your action is only a part of a
great whole of working men, women,
and things, of which you and your reso-
lutions are the smallest fraction. What
you will do depends upon what they
will do and say. This you cannot by
any possibility know, and even if you

could, you are not now in condition to appreciate the bearings of things upon each other and upon you, your power of judgment being in some degree impaired by your isolation. As in the night - obscurity of your chamber you fancy all sorts of threatening and monstrous shapes in articles of furniture or clothing which are very small and harmless, so in the separateness of your excited thought you are really unable to measure and assign their due proportions to arguments and probabilities. The conclusions formulated with so much pains in the night are seen with the first rays of the sun to be of no value in the day-world, and so gradually you learn to save yourself the labor of working them out. As plants are supposed to breathe out a different substance in the dark from that which they exhale by day, so does the human mind by night exhale only impossible fancies.

Learn not to be restless in planning for the future; learn to wait till you come to the bridge before you cross it, and you will be saved many footsteps. Alone in your room, with the uncertainty of the unseen universe around you, and with the fatigue of the day upon you, deprived of any visible or audible standards of measure by which to test the importance of things, you are no more capable of drawing correct conclusions about what you had best do in difficult circumstances than is the hermit in the desert of making out a running schedule for the New York Central Railroad. Charles V. found it difficult to direct the affairs of his kingdom from the monastery of Yuste, and the effort of his restless brain brought him only vexation when, finding weariness in his seclusion, he tried again to take part in the turmoil from which he had fancied he should be glad to escape.

Of course, the more active is the mind, the more difficulty exists in putting it into a state of passivity; teàchers, for instance, whose calling compels them to be active in a high degree on the minds of others, find it at last almost impossible to attain this state; they can teach, but they cannot listen. The incapacity is one of the losses which the profession entails. But, after all, if you are to gain any great amount of good from the world, you must attain a passive condition of mind. He who receives a great many letters demanding answer, sees himself as if engaged in a hopeless struggle of one man against the rest of the world. However, it is never to be forgotten that it is the rest of the world and not you that holds the great share of the world's wealth, and that you must allow yourself to be acted upon by the world, if you would become a sharer in the

gain of all the ages to your own infinite
advantage. Many lose all the possible
benefit to be won by travel because they
have not the necessary passivity. You
should go to picture-galleries and mu-
seums of sculpture to be acted upon,
and not to express or try to form your
own perfectly futile opinion. It makes
no difference to you or to the world
what you may think of any work of art.
That is not the question ; the point is
how it affects you. The picture is the
judge of your capacity, not you of its
excellence; the world has long ago
passed its judgment upon it, and now
it is for the work to estimate you. If
without knowing that a certain picture
is from the hand of a great master, you
find yourself wonderfully affected by it
and drawn to it over and over again, you
may be ·glad that its verdict upon you
is favorable and that you are acquitted
from the possible charge of foolishness,

10

but you ought to be very humble in your gladness. When you go to Cologne Cathedral, sit down and make your mind perfectly passive and empty, and wait for what measure of grace may be vouchsafed to you. In religion the influence which comes to the passive mind— made and held so by the active will— is called Grace, and it is that which will descend upon you in other domains if only you will let it come. The main trouble generally is that by your continual Restlessness you keep your soul in such a state that no influence can come to you from without. And yet from without it is, that all sorts of good things are pressing to reach and to bless you. As a writer in the *Christian Union* says, " No one knows so well as he who does great things how partial and limited is his work, and how divine a refuge from the fragmentariness of his life is absorption in the vastness of

God's work, and obliviousness in the vastness of God's life." But you cannot be absorbed unless you will let yourself be so. One path out of restlessness is by the road of doing great things, which always leads through the valley of humility as it goes, with the kingdom of Heaven at its end.

There is a Restlessness springing from the consciousness of power not fully utilized, which must be present wherever there is unused power of whatever kind. This is the restlessness of the germ within the seed, struggling upward and downward towards its proper life. It is a valuable testimony that there is life within, but where the surroundings are unfavorable, it is a striving full of pain, the cutting of tender flesh by the fetters of the captive as he struggles against their pitilessness. The wild birds that fall dead at the foot of the light-house, dashed back from the

hard glass of the lantern whose light
called them from safe flying in the soft
air, know this. But they fall dead, and
their rest is sudden and swift, while to
the human pain, can be applied only
the palliative of a long patience and
fortitude. But the shadow merely of
Peter healed the sick folk as he passed
by; he did not need even to touch
them with his hand. And so to those
who may have the power for greater
achievement than that for which op-
portunity is granted them, is given the
power to heal by their shadows as they
pass. For the patient self-control, which
goes on bravely in the work possible to
it, while knowing of boundless possibilities unattainable, yields in large measure a harvest of strength felt like the
passing of a strong shadow wherever
it may go. And in knowledge of this
we may find a surcease of the Restlessness with which we seem to ourselves

to be devoured till there is no strength
left. To see power wasted is very hard.
But really no power is ever wasted in
the spiritual kingdom any more than in
the material. It is only transmuted
and correlated, so that there need never
be mourning over a loss which does not
exist, and the Restlessness of mourning
will thus pass over into Rest. It has
been said of an Englishman recently
dead : " As we looked on him and lived
by his side, we knew well that his peculiar grace was worth more, far more,
to the world at large than it could ever
gauge; more, far more, than all the
minor average excellencies that were
strewn thickly around us. . . . No accu-
mulation of lower attainments in the
many could have done for mankind
what this one spiritual achievement ef-
fected by its solitary supremacy. Yet
who could look at it and doubt how
slow had been the process by which it

had been won; how slowly and how
patiently the tree had grown by the wa-
ter-side before, in its due season, it had
brought forth its fruit; the rare grace—
in all the senses of the word 'grace,'
from the highest to the lowest—which
resulted in the fine and subtile courage,
the wise and ingrained humility, of that
vigorous and single mind." When we
bitterly regret our powerlessness, it may
be that we do not trust enough to our

UNCONSCIOUS INFLUENCE.

Drifting dreamily with the tide,
  Slowly away from the sunset's gold,
Leaning over our vessel's side,
  We watched the sail with its drooping fold.

Southward, the slope of a summer hill,
  Strewn with the fragrant, new-made hay;
The horse and hay-wagon waiting still
  For the finished fruit of the sunny day.

The rapid rake, and the gleaming fork
  Tossing its load on the growing pile,
Farmer and wife and children at work
  Sharing the labor, and all the while

One little maiden down on the shore,
　Just where the land and the water meet,
Wandering free till the work was o'er,
　Chasing the waves with gleaming feet,

Singing clearly across the bay,
　All unconscious of listening ear,
Simple ballads, so light and gay,
　We hushed our words as we leaned to hear.

Songs of our school-days long agone,
　Ringing out over the sunset sea;
Then sweet in the silvery childish tone
　The battle-cry for the Land of the Free.

Dreamily drifting by Deer Isle,
　We lay and listened with strange surprise,
Feeling a blessing of peace the while
　Dropping down from the quiet skies;

Feeling our deeper life touched at the core
　By the simple song of the glad child-heart;
And peace in the boat and peace on the shore
　Were so near and yet so far apart!

Living our lives out day by day,
　All unconscious of listening ear,
Singing our song as we go our way,
　Do we know who may be leaning to hear?

Anything is restless which has not a
purpose, and hence it is that listlessness

breeds Restlessness. For listlessness
is really " lustlessness," or pleasureless-
ness — absence of any controlling interest in anything. To be in dead-
earnest about one thing is to be set
free from all sorts of slaveries, and it is
well that the word "lust," or pleasure,
comes from a root meaning to be set
free, or to be released. When Mrs.
Watts Hughes, singing through her ei-
dophone against the disk which vibrated
to the sound, and expecting to see the
lycopodium dust on it take the form
that it had taken before under the
influence of the same tone, found the
particles flying hither and thither, seemingly baffled in their attempts towards
regularity, she did not understand why
this should be so; but she suspected
that she had been singing with too
much force, and upon getting rid of the
over-tones, the obedient dust at once
settled into the beautiful figure she was

looking for. Then she sang against it, pure and true, the *octave* of the note she had given before, and immediately the dust took another figure, the one, as she could now see, between which and the one she had been trying to create, it had before been uncertain, and hence unable to settle upon either. The restlessness of the lycopodium dust was due only to the over-tones. How many of us are singing with over-tones, and wondering why the life-dust is flying hither and thither, and why there is no rest in it? Suppose we were to sing only one pure tone, and see how quickly it would fall into order and symmetry. Or suppose we try an octave higher! The magnetic needle is restless so long as it does not point to the north; but when it does, there is no more Restlessness.

V

BLUE-ROSE MELANCHOLY

HERE is a country, not far off from many of us, where Professor Earle and all those who, like him, are justly anxious as to the fate of the Subjunctive Mood, might lay down all fear, for the speech there has no other mood, except it be the long discredited Potential, or the Conditional of the French and German. This land is full of all perfect things, and has no bad weather, except, now and then, gentle rain on the farms. No plans "gang agley," and to each dweller in it, all the other human beings there have no wills of their own. Railroad trains never miss connection, tele-

grams are never misspelled or wrongly
punctuated, and gas meters are to be
perfectly trusted, as also the companies
that put them in. Good people who
fall into the water always succeed in
reaching land in safety, while all the
bad ones are drowned. The men who
control the government have no other
thought but to direct it properly, and
the citizen may take his ease, free from
any anxiety, even after the Legislature
of his State has resumed its regular
sessions. Riders and drivers always
keep on the right side of the road, and
all the nurses with perambulators are
continually on the watch to see that no
carriage or swiftly galloping horse is
coming upon them. The inhabitants
generally live in beautiful castles after
the Moorish style of architecture, which
are full of all sorts of conveniences,
and never dusty or out of order in any
of their appointments. Abundance of

pure water rises to the top floors in
all of them, and the kerosene used
never smokes. If any repairs are to
be made, the mechanics who have the
work in charge always come in such
succession that no one ever has to take
out the work of another in order to put
in his own; but as a rule there are no
repairs, properly so called, because all
the material used, as also all the work-
manship, is of the first class. The
Irish servants have no cousins, and
the relatives they do have are never
dangerously ill. Children never forget
what is told them to do, and are of
such a nature that they perfectly and
at once understand all the reasons
which influence their elders in giving
directions or issuing prohibitions; this
saves any necessity for explanations,
and prevents disobedience. All school-
teachers, bishops, and fashionable doc-
tors speak the exact truth, and indeed

have no temptation at any time to do otherwise. Trade is absolutely free, and since there is no interference with its regular action, takes care of itself in a perfectly easy way. All the inhab- itants, as might have been expected, are wealthy, and possess perfect health till they die, so that the physicians have very little to do, except to exam- ine, each one, the special organ of the body which he particularly likes, and to write books about it. The authors and publishers live always together in mutual admiration clubs, as do also the actors and the dramatic critics.

This land is not out of sight, though it seems to have been somewhat diffi- cult of access from the earth except to a few who have visited it, and given to it each the name he thought most fit- ting. It is the land of the Blue Rose. When we speak of it, we generally begin our sentences with an "If," and we speak confidently in the future time. The sentences run somewhat after this model : " If this or that were so, I would do thus or so ;" or, "If I had not so much to do, I could be or do so or so." Or generally, " If the here and the now were utterly different from what they are, then I could be quite content ; then I could rest, but as things are, it is quite impossible." The blue rose belongs probably to the same family as the blue flower told of by Novalis, of which Spielhagen says, "That is the flower which mortal eye has never yet seen, and the fragrance of which fills the whole world. Not every creature is delicately enough made to be able to perceive the perfume ; but the night-ingale is intoxicated with it when it sings and sobs and sighs in the moon-light or at early daybreak, and all fool-ish men have been and are drunk with it when they cry in prose or in poetry

to heaven, pouring out their sorrow and
their grief. ... He who has once breath-
ed the perfume of the blue flower has
no more peace and quiet in this life,
but is driven on and on, though his
sore feet pain him, and he yearns to
lay down his weary head to rest. He
asks for a drink at this or that cottage
door, but he returns the emptied cup
without thanks, for there was a fly in
the water, or the cup was not quite
clean, or—well, he was not refreshed
by the drink." We come across the blue
rose again where Sir Thomas Browne
tells us of "a maid of Germany that
lived without meat on the smell of a
rose," but he makes haste to warn us
that she only pretended to be cared for
by God and good angels, and adds that
she was obliged to recant. There is a
gentle melancholy which marks those
who would be quite willing to live if
only they could live in the country where

the blue rose thrives, and which is of so
well-pronounced a type that it is known
by the name that I have ventured to put
at the head of this chapter. It is met in
all classes and ranks of society, and is
especially to be seen in America, probably because the facilities for travel-
ling are here so many and so great
that every one may hope with more or
less degree of confidence to reach the
land at some time, and to spend the
rest of her life in inhaling the perfume
of the blue rose.

How many of us bear about the melancholy of which I speak! How many
a woman is not quite sure that if she
were in altogether different circumstances, she should find no difficulty in
doing all things required of her with
great cheerfulness, if not with positive
joy! She wants to remain a fully grown
bird, but at the same time she blames
fate that she cannot get into the nest

and lie down as she once could. That the nest is not large enough for the old birds, in fact that it was never intended that they should get into it, strikes her as unreasonable. She is always complaining gently that she cannot make her circles squares or her squares circles. She claims all the privileges of a man, and, at the same time, feels hurt if she fail to receive any consideration generally accorded to a woman. She is not at all desirous of a fair field and no favor, but she asks for all the field and all the favor too. She constructs an ideal world out of her own consciousness, and then feels injured because the world around her does not harmonize with it. And thus she falls a victim to blue-rose melancholy.

Sometimes this is because she has too little real work to do; sometimes because she is ignorant of what the world really is. She shuts herself up

11

too much in the narrow circle of her own home and her own folk, and shuns, rather than seeks, contact with other scenes and other classes of people. When she travels she goes in first-class carriages, and at hotels she lives in suites of apartments, with those she knew at home; she changes neither her sky nor her mind. She spends all her winters visiting the same persons and receiving visits from them, and in summer she does the same things and meets the very same people. No wonder that she knows so little of the real world, and thinks it all wrong, and herself a much-abused person because it does not go to suit her; she has a touch of the blue-rose melancholy, and other evils follow in its train. What she wants is the tonic of regular work and enough of it, and the wholesome nervous shock which comes from contact with people entirely different from

herself. Those who are tired from the
strain of long and constant work—even
they could tell her of the tonic effect
of regular and much-demanding labor;
it may be monotonous, and it may become wearying after many years, but it
leaves no time for illness, none for melancholy or for dawdling on lounges,
and none for mind-weariness, which
saps the life and cuts the wrinkles sooner than labor. It is moth and rust that
corrupt.

Only the flowing water is pure and
sweet. Only the spinning top and the
moving bicycle do not fall over. Rest
is not found in irregular and purposeless motion, nor is it stagnation; all
real and firm rest is to be sought in
harmonious action. It is only by constant hewing at the block of marble
that you can find the statue hidden
within it, and it is only by your own
mental activity and decision that you

can determine which of all the possible
statues contained in it you will chisel
out. What difference does it make if, in
shaping your beautiful drinking-fount-
ain, you cut away a hundred tons of
granite from the stone of the quarry,
if so be that at last you shall have a
shapely and well-proportioned work of
art? The best use that could be made
of those tons of granite was to cut them
away and reveal the fountain, and the
work and the weariness, and all the
long years of incompleteness, are not
lost to the life that shapes itself into
beauty and fulfilment at the end there-
of. Go on and make errors, and fall
and get up again. Only go on! You
will never learn to speak a foreign language if you are afraid of mistakes; so
you will never do anything with your
own life if you are discouraged by failure. You were made to fail over and
over again, or you would never gain

any strength. The harder time you
have, the gladder you ought to be; for
you are getting exercise and experience, and, then, God would never spend
so much trouble in training you if you
were not worth the effort. You really
must be of considerable value if you
are turned, twisted, and tried in all
sorts of ways. There was much wisdom in the fable of Antæus; as he
grew stronger by falling, so may you.

Mr. George Nevile, in his *Horses
and Riding*, says, " A man bought a
horse, and after some time was asked
by a friend whether the horse was a
safe horse to ride, on which he replied
that he could not tell, as the horse had
never stumbled with him up to that
time. This was repeated as a good joke,
but is strict sense." It is only one out
of a hundred wise truths which may be
learned from experience with a horse,
for our increase in righteousness.

I saw a squirrel to-day, busy collect-
ing dry leaves. He did not take in-
discriminately, but selected evidently
with much care. He held them by the
stems in his mouth till he had so many
that he looked as if his head were nothing but a bunch of leaves. Then he
made for his nest, which was near the
top of a lofty tree a long distance away;
but he went by circuitous routes, and
at last, when he found a group of children directly in his path, he took to
the trunk of a tree at a considerable distance from his home; on this he climbed
wisely and warily out to the end of a
long branch, then leaped from that to
the end of another on a second tree,
and from that in the same way to his
own, losing, as he did so, one of his
treasures, but not for that reason flinging away the others; then he made
his way, still circuitously, to the nest,
and disappeared in it. Your tasks are

no harder than was his, and you will
have no greater obstacles.   Have you
not his invention and perseverance?
There was no blue-rose melancholy
about him.   And yet his world is a
pretty hard one, considering the existence of human beings in it, and it is
full of all sorts of difficulties.

Can you not

" Be as the bird that chancing to alight
Upon a bough too slight,
Feels it give way beneath her, and yet sings,
Knowing that she hath wings ?"

Your wings must be made of the
same stuff as that from which you have
constructed your melancholy—your own
imagination.   But so long as you think
of nothing but the frailness and the
good-for-nothingness of the bough on
which you have been standing, you will
have no power to use it, even to spring
from.   Take to yourself wings and flee
away.   You think perhaps that the gods

do not care. But if you had read Æschylus you would have learned that "the gods, for what they care for, care enough." And if they do not seem to care for your unequalled trouble, it may be—I say it *may* be—that it is not in their clear eyes worth caring about. It is in reading such writers as Æschylus and not in modern literature that you may often find the antidote for the melancholy which is sapping your strength. A taste for the best literature is a blessed gift; if you have it not yet, strive towards it till you acquire it. Be content to be passive and let yourself be worked upon by it, and finally you may begin to take in its influence actively, and then you will know where to go to find wings, and will flee as a bird to your mountain.

Many people seem to overlook the fact that even Christ and the three disciples did not remain forever on the

Mount of Transfiguration, but came
down again into the low-lying valleys.
Even the hardest days are a component
part of the whole life, and should be
looked at and held as such, not wished
away; there is great force in the conviction that everything that may be in
your life is really a necessary part of it
and cannot be spared, any more than
death can, if it is to be rounded and full.
When you meet trouble and annoyance
in this way, they cease to be enemies
and are changed to friends.   There is
good doctrine in " Aubrey de Vere :"

" Count each affliction, whether light or grave,
    God's messenger sent down to thee ; do thou
    With courtesy receive him ; rise and bow ;
And, ere his shadow pass thy threshold, crave
Permission first his heavenly feet to lave ;
Then lay before him all thou hast ; allow
No cloud of passion to usurp thy brow,
Or mar thy hospitality ; no wave
Of mortal tumult to obliterate
The soul's marmoreal calmness ; Grief should
    be

Like joy, majestic, equable, sedate,
Confirming, cleansing, raising, making free,
Strong to consume small troubles; to com-
    mend
Great thoughts, grave thoughts, thoughts last-
    ing to the end."

The problem before you is unchange-
ably and always, not what you "would
do if "—for that is the way the thought
of blue-rose melancholy runs—but what
you will do on this particular gloomy
day, in this particular room, with the
particular people and things that are in
it. You have got to play the game with
the cards that have been dealt to you,
and it is of no use for you to bewail
your fate because you don't hold different ones. Look them over, arrange
them, and play. You certainly must
play them before you will get any others, and you need never expect to have
other people's cards. You would probably not know how to manage them if
you had them, but that is not the point.

In the land of the blue-rose you would probably have held thirteen trumps, but you are not there, and what is more, you never will get there if you don't play, and play according to the full measure of your ability, the cards you do hold.

"When the armies are set in array, and the
    battle beginning,
  Is it well that the soldier whose post is far
    to the leftward
  Say, 'I will go to the right, it is there I
    shall do best service?'
  There is a great Field - Marshal, my friend,
    who arrays our battalions;
  Let us to Providence trust, and abide and
    work in our stations."

Did you ever read the old proverb which says that it is the same to him whose feet are incased in a shoe as if the whole surface of the earth were covered with leather? Perhaps, after all, you have only to take off your own shoes to find that the ground is not

hard and unyielding, but soft and " re-
sulting " under your tread. At any rate,
the experiment is a simple one; the
hard surface of which you complain
may be only one symptom that you are
falling into blue-rose melancholy.

Your business on this earth is the
same as was that of the Creator at the
first: "the singing of shapeless matter
into symmetry and beauty." Do you
want any higher? But notice that it
is only the singing and not the speaking voice that sends the light lycopodium dust flying into regular forms in
Mrs. Watts Hughes's voice-form exper-
iments. And she warns us that "Success demands considerable practice in
singing, and untiring perseverance in its
employment." Otherwise your chaos
will remain chaos, and your little dust-
heap will be only a little dust-heap at
the end. Who hinders your practice in
singing but yourself?

Blue-rose melancholy, like other sorts of melancholia, is a sympton of insanity, that is, of a want of Reason. It must not be humored, it must be fought. Are there dragons in the road? Attack them! If there is a wall of flame across the path, read the story of Spenser's "Britomart," and then strike spurs into your will and ride at it! That is the only way. But — and this is a great "But"—make yourself sure before you do either, that the dragon and the flames are actually in your road, and not in one of the openings of the impenetrable thicket surrounding the land of the blue rose. If so, the way of discretion as well as the way of valor is to turn back into your actual road again, and not to waste strength by trying to push in thither. You have no right to complain of the roughness of the path if you have voluntarily turned aside from the one assigned you, to climb the wall of a precipice which seemed to lead more directly towards the goal of your wishes; if you have done so, at least have the grace to accept bravely and without murmur what you have yourself chosen. Don't waste time on symptoms when nothing but radical measures will do. Go straight to the root of the matter, to the source of the symptoms. Don't be afraid to recognize that your real trouble is the genuine blue-rose melancholy, and half the battle will have been won.

If you have one continuous thread of some strong purpose in your life, you can disregard things that do not touch it and afford to give them the go-by. Do not waste strength in fighting annoyances which concern not that; then, finally, it may be said of you, as was said of Canon Liddon, that "everything about him was natural and spontaneous, because it was governed by a purpose

so habitual that it was no longer no-
ticed." If you have only a small natural stock of trust, enlist under the ban-
ner of Savonarola and be content to
" live upon the faith of yesterday, waiting for the faith of to - morrow." At
least you can do that, even if you have
no faith to-day, and there are many people who have to live thus, so that you
need not fear to suffer from solitude.
There is the possibility of great virtue
in simply standing still, as well in your
soul as with your body, and there are
many who learn this truth only when it
is too late — if, indeed, there be any
such words as " too late " in the language of God, or any thought which
corresponds to them in His heart.

Walter Pater, in *Marius the Epicurean*,
calls attention to four characteristics of
the Cyrenaic philosophy in which, he
says, " it approached the nobler form of

Cynicism as also the more nobly developed phases of the old or traditional ethics." These are — and they may well give us pause—

"The gravity of its conception of life.

"Its pursuit after nothing less than a perfection.

"Its apprehension of the value of time.

"The passion and the seriousness which are like a consecration."

We live in the light which broke upon the world after the time of these philosophies, but we may well read and reread these words, and ask ourselves how many of the four we have in personal possession. They have been, perhaps, sufficiently illustrated in the preceding chapters of this book, to which they correspond in a somewhat deeper sense than that of mere number.

The demands of modern life consti-

tute the Sphinx of to-day. She has still
all the strength and size of the lion, and
she has still a woman's face.   As of old,
to the answer of the question which
she propounds, there is no alternative
but death, and from answering there is
no escape.

Not only to the Thebans came
The fiery question, winged with flame ;
We hear the same, yet not the same.

Uplifted from her dread domain,
The Sphinx may bring us deathless pain—
Beyond, her threatening is in vain.

I solve no riddle, Sphinx, for thee,
But hold thee fast and rigidly ;
Hope thou for no escape from me.

Not less well-won we count the field
By waiting than by fighting sealed ;
Thou, thou thyself shalt answer yield!

O Life, I hold thee face to face ;
Nor move I back one single pace
For accident of time or space ;

12

For time and space to me belong,
Nor know they how to work me wrong;
I wait, for I, not thou, am strong.

Day after day may slow go by.
After the worst that thou canst try,
At last, at last, thou shalt reply!

No haste—Eternity is now;
No rest—I will not let thee go;
What thou hast asked, that answer *thou!*

THE END.

Breinigsville, PA USA
10 February 2011
255349BV00003B/21/P